Stay Active, Stay Supple, Stay Healthy

Angela Rippon

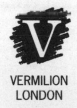

VERMILION
LONDON

First published 1998

1 3 5 7 9 10 8 6 4 2

First published in the United Kingdom in 1998 by Vermilion

an imprint of Ebury Press

Random House UK Ltd
Random House
20 Vauxhall Bridge Road
London SW1V 2SA

Random House Australia (Pty) Ltd
20 Alfred Street, Milsons Point, Sydney,
New South Wales 2061, Australia

Random House New Zealand Limited
18 Poland Rd, Glenfield,
Aukland 10, New Zealand

Random House, South Africa (Pty) Limited
Endulini, SA Jubilee Road, Parktown 2193, South Africa

Random House UK Limited Reg. No. 954009

A CIP catalogue record for this book is available from the British Library.

ISBN 0 09 186267 1

Typeset in New Baskerville by Clive Dorman & Co.

Printed and bound in UK by Caledonian International, Bishopbriggs

Papers used by Vermilion are natural, recyclable products made from wood grown in sustainable forests.

Contents

Introduction

Staying healthy and active is an option that's now open to more and more of us even when we've hit that time of life that some people persist in calling 'middle age'...

I've reached my fifties, it's no secret! But I can honestly say I haven't really noticed any slowing down or any loss of energy. It's partly the attitude I notice in my friends and family. We don't let the fact we're getting older make much of a difference to what we wear, how we enjoy ourselves or the activities we get involved in.

I know I'm luckier than some. I've inherited some healthy genes and I have never yet had to cope with prolonged or serious ill health. I've broken my nose three times! And I once broke both my arms in a riding accident. But I made a good recovery each time. Yet it's not just the fact that I'm basically healthy that keeps my energy levels up. I also try to make sure I fit in some daily stretching exercises wherever I am and, as you'll see as you read through, I enjoy other activities as well.

This book will give you plenty of ideas to inspire you to take more exercise without making it a chore. The 28-day exercise plan will give you results you can see and feel, but you don't have to stick to the stretching and moving we suggest. In fact, brisk walking, gardening, golfing or even dancing can do you just as much good if you keep it up and put enough zest into it.

The point is to do something you enjoy. We're all human, there's only so much we can put up with if we're not getting much pleasure out of it. No one pays you to exercise, or forces you to do it. It's all down to you. It's voluntary, and the health benefits are hidden, at least at first, before you start to realise how much fitter and more energetic you are. It can actually feel like hard work in the very first few days and finding time in a busy life can be a problem. No wonder we tend to give up if we find the actual activity boring or unrewarding. My advice is to find something you really like doing and stick at it, enjoying the sensation of becoming truly *good* at it as time goes on.

In my work, no two weeks are the same. But I have my share of hours sitting at my desk in front of a computer screen, writing and researching scripts, and I do a fair amount of travelling by car, train and plane. I can see why some people with a desk-bound job, or people who have to drive around in a car from job to job, can get out of the habit of regular exercise.

In the media there are plenty of people who seem to thrive on pressure, but who wind down after a stressful day with several drinks and yet more sitting around. I admit I like a certain amount of pressure. I love getting involved in new projects, coming up with new ideas and seeing teamwork bring them to fruition beating dead-lines along the way. And of course it's important to relax whenever things feel as if they're piling up. But I've recognised that as you get older, it's even more impor-tant to relax in the right way. And for me that includes exercising, though I must admit I do like a glass of cham-pagne occasionally. I think it does me good.

When I was a child, I learnt to dance and a love of dance has stayed with me all my life. I still use dance movements I learnt over 12 years or so to keep me supple, perhaps that's why I'm more flexible than a lot of people my age. I hate feeling stiff and creaky and not able to move as quickly as I want to because of twinges, so I keep up my stretches as a routine. I certainly know when I've missed doing them.

A few years ago I discovered for myself how changing your diet can make you feel better. I'd been suffering from headaches and stomach pains which didn't seem to have anything to do with any underlying illness. In the end, I saw a nutritionist who investigated dietary causes. She put me on an exclusion diet, which meant I was eating a very basic diet for a few weeks. Then we started to introduce other foods and noted when the symptoms began. In this way, we found out that I should avoid dairy produce, anything which contained wheat and red wine. It may sound difficult, but believe me, it's not – and it certainly pays off. I've discovered things like soya, and pasta, made from rice and buckwheat, and goat and sheep yoghurts and cheese. Non-dairy ice cream is pretty good, too.

I stick to a mainly healthy, low-fat diet as well as avoiding my 'no no' foods. Eating healthily doesn't mean eating foods you don't like, or using weird and unobtainable ingredients. The recipes in this book have all been selected for their ease, all the ingredients are widely available, and all the dishes are quick and simple to prepare. They taste good, too, which is just as important.

I use supplements as a way of ensuring that my body gets the nutrients it needs and to keep my energy levels up. You can read more about these on page 108. There are times when we cannot guarantee that our diet is balanced enough to supply everything, and as there's a lot of evidence that the right supplements can help maintain good health, taking them every day makes sense to me. I'm especially impressed with cod liver oil. I was given a dose every day at nursery school laced with orange juice to make it taste better! My, hasn't it come a long way since then! It's fascinating – and encouraging – to see how something that's been so well known for generations really is recognised by science as a valuable source of nutrients.

Do enjoy reading the book and enjoy an active, supple, healthy life!

Angela Rippon

Section One
STAY ACTIVE

Introduction

Here's where we look at the whole process of ageing and it's something scientists still don't fully understand. Are we all 'programmed' from birth to age at a specific rate? Probably not, though inheritance plays a part. Can we change the rate we age by changing the way we live, work, play and eat? It looks like it. Which is the most important element in the health equation? We don't know, though it seems from research that staying active can go some way to combat the undoubted ill-effects of being overweight and eating the sort of diet that we know has an adverse effect on health.

Ageing, fitness and health are areas that involve a range of medical and social specialities, and there has been a veritable explosion of research in the last generation. We report on just a small selection of it here, it makes interesting reading! This section also challenges your knowledge of the answers so far and we look at ways of staying mentally active as well.

Angela Rippon

Chapter One
Getting On in Years ... and Slowing Down?

To our great-grandparents, and even our grandparents, the very idea that you might remain energetic and active in your middle years and beyond would have been strange.

While getting older and maybe succumbing to the illnesses and physical conditions we associate with ageing can't have been welcome to anyone at any time in history, it's only recently that many of us have begun to question whether 'slowing down' is inevitable and whether we can enjoy being physically active as long as we want to. Is remaining active totally outside our control? Is it just a matter of luck and the genetic background we've inherited? Or can we affect our chances of staying as close as possible to peak physical condition, continuing to take part in the sports and other activities we enjoyed as younger people, and resisting any aches and pains that might put the brakes on?

It's an important question. After all, half of us are likely to live into our late seventies and eighties and even beyond. If at all possible, we want to enjoy the extra couple of decades that the combined efforts of improved medicine, sanitation, health, nutrition and knowledge have handed to us this century!

Why Do We 'Get Older' as We Age?

Medical and biological, and more recently biochemical, research has long asked why all of us, no matter how healthy we may be for most of our lives, exhibit at least some signs of ageing. Some of the theories that still have at least partial credibility with today's experts include:

- the idea that all the body's cells simply suffer wear and tear, and eventually degenerate and cease to function through use
- the idea that the body's cells have an 'in-built' and unchangeable limit to the number of divisions they can undergo before they start to break down and eventually stop working
- the idea that the body ceases to be able to repair damaged DNA in its cells because of the effect of free radicals *(see below)*

New research has identified that certain rogue molecules (free radicals) contribute to cell damage, which may be one explanation for the ageing process.

Free radicals circulate in every part of our body. We can't avoid producing them, as they are the natural result of bodily processes such as breathing. It's thought they have a positive function in helping fight infection. However, they can and do attack and damage other cells in the body, and overloading the body with 'excess' free radicals speeds up this damage. Excess free radicals come at us from the environment, from pollution, from sunlight, and from our own intake of pollutants, for example in foods and in cigarettes. Somehow, the healthy young body is able to 'mop them up', reducing the number of free radicals to within the limits of the body's ability to cope. As we get older, though, it is thought that the body is less able to deal with the excess free radicals.

Is It All Inevitable?

Despite some headline-grabbing adventures with real people, scientists are still discussing exactly how to limit the damage of free radicals and just how effective limitation can be. At some point, it seems, ageing and its consequent 'slowing down' are unavoidable. For example, for most of us there is an increase in body fat after about 45 and a consequent decrease in muscle mass. Our bones get thinner and there is a higher risk of fractures. Our lung and heart functions slow, so we get 'puffed out' more quickly than before when undertaking anything out of the ordinary in the way of physical activity.

The good news is that these changes can be slowed down by taking physical exercise – and while the sooner you start the better, leaving it late is no excuse for not bothering!

The trouble is, it's not as easy as simply making a resolution to change. Getting into the habit – often the brand new habit – of exercise is the hardest part of it. The way you live your life can drastically reduce your motivation for getting started and then continuing. But there's almost always an answer to your objections!

Exercise – for Everyone!

John's problem:

At 48, John's reached a level of responsibility at work where he feels required to be first at his desk in the

morning and last to go at night. 'My work is stimulating
and invigorating,' he says, 'and I enjoy it. I really can't
see how I'd find the time to take exercise – yet I know I
should. I take the stairs instead of the lift when I can,
but that's about it.'

Possible solutions:

- John can cycle to and from work on days when he
  doesn't need the car there, taking a clean shirt with
  him and leaving a business suit, tie and shoes to
  change into in his office cupboard.
- He can get up half an hour earlier three or four times
  a week and enjoy some brisk walking or jogging.
- He can join a gym which opens long hours, so he can
  choose to visit either before work or afterwards, or, if
  there's a gym or a swimming pool near his office, he
  can make sure he spends some lunchtimes there.

Mary's problem:

Mary, 53, has been plagued with a 'bad back' since a car
accident some years ago. Doctors have advised her to
avoid strenuous exercise or anything which puts a strain
on her lower back. Even walking for more than a short
distance produces an ache which stays with her all day. 'I
hate the way my waistline keeps on spreading, but what
can I do?' she says. 'I feel unfit and lazy, but I don't want
to do myself any damage.'

Possible solutions:

- Mary can try swimming – it gives a great full-body
  work-out and tones all muscle groups, yet it won't put
  a strain on Mary's back as it is not a weight-bearing
  exercise. She can start slowly and build up to a challenging pace.

- What about yoga? Mary needs to find a qualified teacher who can let her know which postures she can do safely and comfortably.
- An assessment by an osteopath or chiropractor might help Mary's back pain and allow her to become more active without suffering pain.

Julia's problem:

Julia has always been overweight, right from a child. She says she's 'allergic to exercise' as it has so many unpleasant memories for her. At school she was laughed at because she couldn't keep up with the other girls at netball and hockey, and PE was no fun either, as she hated the way she looked in shorts. Diets have come and gone throughout her adult life, and now, at 45, she says she's resigned to being fat. She's tired of having lost and then regained the same two stone all the way through her adult life – and it becomes more and more difficult to lose each time. She would like to feel fitter, but she can't think of any exercise she'd actually enjoy doing. 'I've tried exercise classes, but by the time the next week comes round, I've lost heart,' she says.

Possible solutions:

- 'Yo-yo dieting' – where the weight comes on and off repeatedly – is not good for Julia's overall health, and if she is not seriously overweight, staying happy may well be better for her, as long as she's no couch potato. Working on feeling good about herself at last may also help her gain the confidence to exercise in a group or by herself.
- Some fitness centres and gyms have classes for larger people – a ring round locally will give her some options.

- She could try something completely new to go with her new outlook. How about ballroom dancing or line dancing? Gaining a new skill at the same time as exercising is fun, and may well increase her motivation to stay with it!

Bob's problem:

Bob is 74 and has undergone surgery to replace both his arthritic knee joints. This has improved his life, as he is no longer in pain every day. However, he says he has got out of the habit of regular exercise, especially since his dog died and he no longer has to walk every day. He feels overweight and slow, and as a widower is lonely and unwilling to take part in group activities. Yet his doctor has suggested he start exercising to keep his joints and muscles working. 'I don't see what there is for me to do,' he says. 'I don't have the cash to join expensive classes.'

Possible solutions:

- If Bob still suffers from the pains of arthritis elsewhere, his physiotherapist can advise him on regular stretching exercises to both help his current condition and to prevent it getting worse. This might sound boring and even uncomfortable, but a few minutes a day may be all he needs.
- Local leisure centres often have reduced rates for older people, either for membership or one-off classes, as well as special facilities for them. It can take courage to go along to somewhere new if you've always been used to living life as a couple, but taking the plunge is worthwhile (and remember that most people in a class are there on their own).
- Swimming is excellent for someone like Bob, as he

can do it at his own pace, and it is perfect for people with mobility problems.
- Why not get another dog?

Keep It Up!

Remember, exercise doesn't have to be strenuous or fatiguing to have an effect, but it does have to be regular and a permanent fixture in your life!

Aim to build up to exercising three to five times a week, for half an hour each time. Anything which challenges you without exhausting you is fine! In order to gain some benefit, you have to feel as if you've *worked!*

Turn to page 61 for our suggested fit-in-a-month exercise plan, which you can begin any time, even if you haven't exercised for years.

Check your Progress!

You can do a simple test to see how fit you are and what effect your extra activity is having on your all-round body 'performance'.

Stand at the foot of your stairs and step on and off the bottom stair continuously for three minutes. Don't go mad – take about two seconds to complete each step. Then stop and assess the level of difficulty, on a scale of say one to five, where five is very difficult or virtually impossible, and one is easy.

If you are very fit, you'll score one or two.
If you are moderately fit, you'll score three.
If you are unfit, you'll score four or five.

continued overleaf

Aim to up your fitness one, two or even three notches. If you are healthy, without any underlying joint problems, and not very overweight, this should be possible after some weeks of regular exercise.

Bodies and Machinery

'Years ago, I interviewed Eileen Fowler,' says Angela. 'She's best remembered as one of the leading lights of the League of Health and Beauty – many people over 50 and 60 will remember that, I'm sure. She was also one of the very first people to bring the idea of healthy exercise to the TV audience. She told me her philosophy was that the body was just like a machine – and if you don't use every bit of it, it stops working efficiently.'

Angela has also met many athletes and dancers over the years. 'I've always been impressed by the way they respect their bodies and treat them with care. That way, of course, their bodies work better, for longer.'

Birthday Splash

How about splashing out on your birthday – with exercise? When Elsie Holden from Bingham, near Nottingham, hit 70, she decided to forgo the party and the presents. Instead, she swam a celebratory 70 lengths of her local pool. With sponsorship from her friends in place of gifts, she raised a grand total of £500 for young homeless people. She's now planning to do 80 lengths in 10 years' time!

Stay Cool!

The older you get, the more important it is to cool down

with a few stretches after exercise – that way you prevent stiffness and discomfort the next day and ensure you get the full benefit from your exercise.

Wind Down

As well as cooling down, always slow down gradually when you come to the end of your aerobic exercise – suddenly stopping could make you feel faint.

Too Old?

Never think you're too old to exercise. In fact, once you hit 30, say the experts, you're too old *not* to exercise!

Don't think that because you were a sporty person when you were younger that now, after possibly decades of inactivity, you're still fit. Unfortunately, you can't store up fitness in that way. The truth is that muscle starts to waste if it isn't used and you can lose aerobic fitness after just two or three weeks. The good news is you *can* get that strength and fitness back again.

Weight Watching?

There's no doubt that exercising is an important part of any weight-loss programme and staying active can help keep you trim without you even thinking much about it. Some people are naturally slender, but it's as well not to take that natural tendency for granted.

Angela Rippon says she is happy with her weight at present. 'It's about nine stone, and though that's rather more than I weighed in my 20s, I feel okay with it.

Fortunately, my weight seems to stay the same without me having to pay much attention to it. I weigh myself at the gym every so often, just to check.'

Muscling In

According to the Central YMCA (the international organisation devoted to the development of mind, body and spirit, and renowned for its research into fitness), older muscle shows just the same potential to improve as younger muscle. In one study at London's Royal Free Hospital women aged 75 to 93 were helped to start exercising their muscles and their progress was followed over 12 weeks. They all managed to increase their muscle strength, some by up to 30 per cent. So it's never too late!

Work Out your Weight

The best way to decide if you need to lose weight is to look in the mirror, rather than at the scales. If you're honest, you can tell whether you look larger than you'd like to be.

A more 'scientific' way to work out whether you need to lose weight is to know your BMI, or body mass index. This gives you a wide range of 'normal' and takes into account your height (though not your age).

To work out your BMI, you need to have your height in metres and your weight in kilograms. Now, multiply your height by itself to gets its square and divide your weight by the answer. The formula is:

$$\frac{\text{WEIGHT (kg)}}{\text{HEIGHT (m) x HEIGHT (m)}}$$

What's the resulting number?

- If it's under 20, you're underweight.
- If it's between 20 and 25, you are fine, and at a healthy weight.
- If it's between 26 and 30, you're overweight.
- If it's over 30, you are seriously overweight and need to seek advice on losing at least some weight for your health's sake.

Note: If you are very lean and very muscular, with very little body fat (like a body builder), the BMI is not very useful. You may appear to be overweight on the score and yet in reality you aren't.

Keep It in the Family

'I think I'm lucky to come from a healthy family,' says Angela. 'We've always been active, and my father and mother, who are 78 and 76, are both very fit. My dad often goes hiking on Dartmoor for the day – he's away six hours sometimes!'

Getting Started

You can exercise anywhere, any time, but many people find actually joining a club and/or a class keeps up their motivation. These days, gyms and fitness centres are working desperately hard to get rid of their 'posers in Lycra' image. Expensive, upmarket places may cling to that idea, but far more places realise that most of us are pretty ordinary and don't want to go to a gym to show off! And if we're somewhere where there are other people who do seem to be concerned about their appearance and performance, we feel more than a mite uncomfortable. That's why you might be pleasantly surprised by visiting a centre these days. Staff are concerned to put you at your ease, and most will devise an exercise programme for you, tailor-made to take into account your available time, any underlying conditions which affect how you exercise and any specific needs you tell them about.

Cost may be a factor. Generally speaking, local authority-owned centres are likely to be slightly cheaper than private places, though the facilities may not be so good. Most places, private and public, have special rates for people of pensionable age, and you may be able to get special off-peak rates, whatever your age, if you can visit during the day.

Don't Be Squashed!

One of the greatest motivators for continuing an active life is to be with people whose company you enjoy and to feel you have mastered a new physical challenge.

Learning to play a sport in later life fits the bill twice over. Take squash. At top level, it's a hard, fast game that demands a lot in the way of stamina, strength and endurance. But because of these very qualities, it gives the mind and body a wonderful work-out – even if you play at a much lower level.

Egyptian-born squash professional Moussa Halel is 49 and now based at a fitness centre near Manchester. He is regularly ranked in the world top 3 for the over 40s. Now

UK-based, he spends much of his time teaching squash to older people. 'Squash is a wonderful game for all ages. I find anyone can play it – I regularly coach people over 60 who have never picked up a squash racket in their lives.'

Squash is a demanding sport and probably not advisable for you if you haven't exercised for a while. But once you have reached a certain level of fitness and flexibility, have a go!

Angela's Exercise Routine

Angela belongs to a gym which is just a few blocks away from her home in central London. 'I try to go at least once a week,' she says, 'and I often manage more than this, depending on my work schedule. I also do a yoga class once a week.'

Her routine at the gym is fairly standard. 'I do half an hour's power walking on the treadmill, followed by 15 minutes or so on the weights machines. Then I finish off with 15 to 20 lengths of the pool.'

She also has a daily routine of stretching, which she does as soon as she gets up. 'I feel I've got my body into gear, then, and I'm ready for the day. I do 40 sit ups, plus stretches for back, neck, hips and shoulders. I notice that if I miss out this routine I get the odd twinge and that reminds me I need to get back to it.'

Angela learnt this routine, or the basis of it, when she was a child taking dancing lessons. 'I really feel it's a good way to get the body aligned – it's a bit like a cat, stretching after being asleep.'

You can find our suggested stretching routine on page 52.

Get Approval First

Most of the exercise advocated in this book is perfectly safe for anyone to do, at any age. However, if you have any doubts at all about your health, about any past or present injuries or disabilities, or about your weight, see your doctor first if you are unused to exercise. Tell him or her the sort of programme you intend to do and get his or her approval. This could actually increase your motivation – telling your doctor of changes you're about to make for your health will probably make you more likely to stick at your programme.

Ouch!

If you're unlucky enough to hurt yourself as a result of exercise (or anything else), don't continue with your activity. Seek medical advice if the pain doesn't go away and avoid exercising in that particular way until your injury has healed. It's possible you've stretched a ligament beyond its elasticity or put too much pressure on a joint.

Never exercise through pain.

Slow Down...

Stop your exercise if:

- your pulse rate becomes irregular
- you feel dizzy or faint
- you feel pain
- you become unusually short of breath compared to what you are used to with this form of exercise

You're doing too much if:

- you take more than five minutes to recover from an exercise session – that is, you're still sitting or lying with a racing heart and suffering breathlessness after you've finished
- you often feel sick after exercise
- you feel stiff and uncomfortable the next day, despite cooling down

Swim Right!

Swimming is a good form of exercise for everyone, but be careful how you do it. You can suffer lower back and neck strain if your technique is at fault.

First, check you're holding yourself correctly. Too many people hold their head out of the water as they don't want water on their face or in their eyes. This causes unnecessary strain and that can lead to injury. Putting your head in the water for each stroke improves your breathing and makes the exercise you get with swimming more effective. Buy some efficient swimming goggles that don't let in water, so your eyes don't sting afterwards.

You can't totally avoid getting your hair wet, but a well-fitting cap will go some way towards keeping the worst of the water off. If you find swimming-pool water is bad for your hair's condition, rub some conditioner into your hair before swimming and then wash it out under the shower afterwards. It has to be said, though, that elaborate hairstyles probably don't go with regular swimming.

Small Steps, Big Changes

As well as making space in your life to take on a more regular, planned exercise programme, smaller changes can add up to a real difference. Don't groan when you hear some of them – you'll have read them or heard them from other people many times before, but that doesn't make them any less valuable.

• Never take the lift if you can walk upstairs. OK, if you live or work on the eighth floor, you may want to take the lift as a rule. But just occasionally, why not try to cope without?
• Get off the train or bus sooner than usual and walk the rest of way.
• Walk to the shops and take the bus back.
• If you use your car a lot, use a car park further away than you normally do.
• Visiting friends nearby for a social evening? Walk there and back in your trainers or comfortable shoes, taking your smart shoes with you to change into.

Dance Away!

Angela Rippon learnt to dance as a child – and who can forget that wonderful appearance on *The Morecambe and Wise Show* where she stunned the nation with her high-kicking grace? Later, of course, she continued her association with dance in the public mind by presenting BBC TV's *Come Dancing*.

'I never trained as a professional dancer,' she says, 'but the love of dance has stayed with me. I think it's a wonderful way to keep fit and lithe. It's great to see all forms of dancing being enjoyed by so many people.'

Dance is a wonderful tonic for body and mind, and gives an excellent aerobic work-out, too. You don't have to stick to the traditional forms of dance – there are dozens available today and your local library will have information about classes.

The Line Dancers

Pat, 72, and Jack, 71, tried line dancing for the first time as part of an evening organised by their local Rotary Club. Line dancing is literally done in a line. You follow the moves shown to you by the caller, and it involves a lot of whole-body movement and co-ordination.

Pat says, 'It was wonderful. I'd definitely do it again. It didn't matter that I hadn't a clue about the steps at first. You just watch the caller, copy the person in front of you and hope for the best! It was a lot of fun and I really felt I'd had some good exercise.'

Chapter Two
What's your Activity Score?

Try this quiz and test your knowledge of the body's functioning, and the effects and benefits of an active life. Intelligent guesses are perfectly acceptable if you're not certain of your answers! Actually doing the quiz will help you learn more about exercise, too.

1. Someone who exercises regularly is less likely to have high blood pressure than someone who takes very little exercise.
    True/False
2. The fitter you are, the longer it takes to 'push' your heart rate upwards during exercise.
    True/False
3. Aerobic exercise should be short in duration and very intense in order to have maximum effect.
    True/False
4. The main purpose of non-aerobic exercise is to develop strength and power.
    True/False
5. Underline the types of exercise which are aerobic:
    Swimming; running; scuba diving; weight training; cycling; yoga; dancing; rowing
6. A calorie is a measure of fat in your food.
    True/False

7. Exercise needs to be uncomfortable to be effective.
   True/False
8. Gardening and DIY can be just as effective exercise as swimming or cycling.
   True/False
9. How much work does your heart have to do each day? It pumps how many gallons of blood…
   a) *1,000*
   b) *2,000*
   c) *4,000*
10. Some exercise could make you more susceptible to illness than before.
    True/False
11. As we get older, our daily diet should have fewer calories.
    True/False
12. Three lots of 10-minutes' exercise is as good as 30 minutes on the trot.
    True/False
13. You shouldn't exercise every day. Your body needs a rest in order to restore itself.
    True/False
14. Your heart quite naturally slows down as you get older.
    True/False

Here are the answers. How did you do?

1. *True*. Blood pressure reflects the work your heart is undertaking simply to keep your circulation going. Unfit people's hearts have to work harder just to keep in action at all, and if your heart is constantly working harder than normal, it can cause damage to the heart itself, to the arteries and to other major

bodily organs. That's why high blood pressure can be a precursor of heart disease. A rise in blood pressure seems to be an inevitable part of growing older, though some researchers feel diet and lifestyle have an important role to play. Regular exercise has been shown to maintain a normal blood pressure, and in some cases it can lower blood pressure and normalise cholesterol levels (cholesterol is the fat that can line the circulatory system and make circulation sluggish).

2. *True*. It makes sense – if you're not fit and unused to exercise, a short run for the bus will puff you out, as it will only take a short time to get your heart up to 'challenge' level. As you become more active and fitter, you can run for longer without giving up. Stairs aren't so much of an effort and you find you're less likely to be breathless after sudden, unexpected exercise. If you are new to exercise, this may be the first positive benefit you notice.

However, remember good effective exercise for all-round fitness does not push you to the limits. Instead, it gets you to a point where you are working your heart more than normal, but not overworking it. Your 'training zone' is calculated at 60–80 per cent of your maximum heart rate *(see also question 14)*.

3. *False*. Aerobic exercise – the sort that gets you slightly out of breath and which targets general body fitness – is most effective done moderately, and for at least 20–30 minutes at a time. Two lots of 10 minutes with a rest in between are not so good!

4. *False*. Non-aerobic exercise does this, focusing on the strength and endurance of particular muscle groups, and improving the suppleness and flexibility of the joints. For all-round health and fitness, you need to

do both types of exercise.

5. The aerobic forms of exercise are swimming, running, cycling, dancing and rowing. Anything which you can maintain for several minutes at a continuous level is deemed to be aerobic.

6. *False*. A calorie is a measure of energy.

7. *False*. Warming up and cooling down before and after any exercise *(see pages 65 and 77)* will prevent discomfort, and any actual pain should be avoided. However, there is a not entirely unpleasant all-over 'ache' you might feel after extra effort and energy output, but it should leave you feeling refreshed, not uncomfortable. Real stabs of pain or even twinges should be a signal to slow down or stop.

8. *True* – but only if your gardening and DIY are hard work! Digging, for example, is pretty taxing, as are painting and papering. But genteel snipping or occasional picture hanging don't count as an exercise programme!

9. c)

10. *True*. Studies have shown that marathon runners are more susceptible to some respiratory infections, for example, and over-exertion can tax the body, causing injury and strain.

11. *True*, unfortunately. It's estimated that for every five years over the age of 25, we actually need 50 fewer calories a day to stay at the same weight, because of the way our metabolic rate (the way we process and use the food we eat) tends to change, and possibly because we tend to become less active as we age. It's not only very common, but is actually normal to weigh more in middle age than in youth. This is not necessarily unhealthy (unless you were already overweight in your 20s), as long as you are fit and active.

12. *False,* although three lots of 10 minutes are better than no exercise at all and in research do show benefits. Also, if you're unused to exercise, you may not be able to manage more than 10 minutes at a time. However, you will reap more rewards if you make the effort to exercise without a break for that half hour – it's the continuous nature of the exercise that gives your heart and lungs the real challenge.

13. *False* – unless you are exercising very intensively, aiming to increase muscle strength and endurance, when time for repair and restoration is normally built into the schedule. Moderate exercise, focusing on stretching and aerobic activity, with no gruelling muscle work, can be done by most people every day.

14. *True,* but you wouldn't be aware of it. The maximum heart rate – that's the number of beats per minute when you are exercising to the absolute limit of your powers – reduces over the years. A 30-year-old is normally reckoned to have a maximum heart rate of 190; at 60, this figure falls to 160 (it's calculated as 220 minus your age). As you get older, your heart also takes progressively longer to get back to its normal resting rate after exercise.

Chapter Three
Your Healthy, Active Life

You can make a real difference to your health, your outlook and your future well-being if you decide now to inject some more physical activity into your everyday routine.

Here are just some of the benefits proven by research:

- Exercise makes you feel good. After 10 minutes of sustained exercise, the body releases the hormone epinephrine. This hormone promotes a general feeling of happiness.
- Exercise improves circulation.
- Tasks requiring mental aptitude are performed better and more accurately after a period of exercise, compared with before.
- Older people who undergo regular aerobic exercise show more mental alertness in tests compared to people in their peer group who do no exercise – possibly because of the improved blood flow to the brain.
- Women who have gone through or who are going through the menopause are less likely to develop osteoporosis if they do regular weight-bearing exercise. This sort of exercise helps retain bone mass and counters the tendency for the bones to weaken as we age.
- People living inactive lives are at a greater risk of

stroke – and the risk is reduced according to the level of your physical activity. A 'sedentary lifestyle' in middle age almost doubles your risk of stroke, compared to people leading 'active' lives. Research also shows that exercise reduces the risk of a second stroke in patients who have already suffered one.

- Exercise helps with digestive problems such as irritable bowel syndrome and constipation, both very common in our later years.
- Feelings of calm after exercise last two to four hours, according to research, once it's a routine. These effects were noted after exercise had been going on for four weeks, but not before.
- Aerobic exercise such as walking reduces the risk of developing heart disease, which can lead to heart attack.
- Regular exercise can help control your weight, by burning off excess fat.
- Joints and tendons remain well-lubricated and more flexible with regular activity.
- Exercise affects your general outlook, doing wonders for self-esteem and confidence. Taking on new activities and learning new routines are especially beneficial if you feel life is in danger of passing you by as you get older.
- Exercise can improve your social life and bring about psychological benefits as a result. Joining a class, a club or a team may be difficult if you're shy, but most people enjoy introducing newcomers to their interests and welcome those who join on their own.
- Exercise reduces fatigue – the pleasant feeling of tiredness after a challenging exercise session is not the same as the day-in day-out fatigue experienced by so many of us today.

- Exercise is an important stress reliever – you can empty your mind of all the thoughts racing through your head, or else allow the break away from your hectic life to give yourself time to 'sort things out'.
- Muscle strength and co-ordination in older people are improved with regular exercise, which in turn protects against falls and injuries.

Exercise for Health

The charity Research into Ageing says exercise is almost as important as not smoking in its overall health benefits.

Angela has never been a smoker. 'Never been tempted,' she says. 'In fact, I feel uncomfortable if I'm somewhere where there's a lot of smoke. It makes my eyes water and it can affect my voice – which if you're presenting on TV or radio is not a good thing.'

Sleep Well

Some people find they sleep a lot better at night once they start exercising regularly.

A Royal Success Story

The King of Tonga, Taufa'ahau Tupou IV, is a prime example of exercise leading to improved health. A few years ago, doctors feared he would have a stroke or develop severe heart disease as a result of his weight (32 stone) and his lack of activity. He was in his mid-70s and already had dangerously high blood pressure. The king didn't want to go on a punishing 'slimming' diet; instead he ordered his aides to come up with a regime that allowed him to indulge his rather more than healthy appetite yet still lose weight and regain what health he could.

The answer was exercise.

These days, the king makes daily visits to the gym. He jogs. He cycles. He swims. He rows. He lifts weights. His programme had to be tailor-made to take into account the fact that his heart and his joints were already working close to capacity just in hauling him around. But after a short time, his heart rate showed signs of improvement and his blood pressure came down. Ever so slightly smaller portions of food and a very small reduction in the fat content of his favourite dishes meant that his diet had a role to play in the changes. But the main change was in his level of activity.

In 1997, after two years on his exercise programme, His Majesty weighed 24 stone. He confidently predicts further weight loss and plans to have come down to 18 stone by the year 2001. His success has inspired an island-wide anti-obesity campaign.

Set your Targets

You may decide that 'getting fit' or 'fitter' is a sufficient goal, but being more specific will make any upsurge in activity more effective, as you'll monitor your progress more closely and maintain your enthusiasm once you see the benefits.

Here's what you might do:

- Need to lose weight? Be realistic – supermodel weights are neither possible nor desirable. Instead, you may decide to move from 'very overweight' to 'slightly

overweight', or just to lose a stone or two.
- Divide your weight loss into segments of five pounds and give yourself a treat when you achieve each step. (*Note:* You can achieve weight loss with exercise alone, but it's likely to be slower than if you combine it with a change in your eating patterns.)
- Don't weigh yourself more than once a week at the most. It takes at least that long for change to show up on the scales. A weight loss of one to two pounds a week is fine. Use scales you can rely on, so you don't cheat yourself that any gain or plateau-ing is the fault of the scales, not you!
- If your blood pressure is high, ask your doctor for a sensible level to target. Return for checking every three months, or when your doctor advises.
- Aim to work up to exercising a fixed number of times per week, for a fixed time each session. You can follow our four-week programme *(see pages 61–87)* or devise your own.

Challenge yourself, but be realistic. Small, gradual changes are likely to be longer lasting than dramatic changes that wear you out and whose novelty value diminishes very quickly. Suddenly throwing yourself into exercise can increase the risk of injury too.

Section Two
STAY SUPPLE

Introduction

There are few things more frustrating if you've been used to your body doing everything you tell it to do than finding things don't 'work' quite as smoothly as they should. Aches and pains and restricted mobility can arise for a number of reasons but in many cases you can improve matters, and this section tells you how.

You'll find the exercise programme on page 61 is something of a challenge if it's been some while since you took regular exercise, but it won't hurt, we promise! The biggest change might be getting into the habit of just doing it... But if you keep it up, you'll feel more energetic, more supple and pretty pleased with yourself as well.

The exercises are devised so that you can make progress and feel you're doing so, day by day, week by week. You'll see, and feel, how you can stretch that bit further and keep going that bit longer.

Don't feel you need to stick to our ideas. They're there to get you going. The best form of exercise is one you enjoy for its own sake. One of my own favourites is yoga. I would hate to have to give that up, as I feel it brings me all-round benefits in mental and physical health.

Angela Rippon

Chapter Four
Moving, Bending, Lifting, Stretching...!

Being supple is a health benefit we take for granted when we're children or young adults. Reaching up for something on a high shelf, bending down to pick something up off the floor, stepping on and off a bus without a thought – and of course, being able to undertake the general exercise that's so beneficial to heart and lung health and well-being... It's all so easy then!

Reason? The bones of the skeleton, the joints, tendons and ligaments and muscles are in tip-top order, obeying our body's impulses by moving as freely as they need to.

A Brief Look at the Body

Bones change as we age, becoming more dense until the mid-30s and then, because they lose calcium (their main component), they start to thin. This process is more marked in women after the menopause, as a response to the drop in oestrogen levels.

Repeated exercise or work can, however, actually build bone – X-rays of tennis players show the arm that holds the racket is thicker than the other one, for example – and with regular exercise bone density can increase even after the thinning process has begun.

Joints are either 'hinge' types, such as where the bones of the arm contact each other at the elbow, or ball-and-socket structures, whereby the rounded end of one bone (such as the thigh) rolls around the hollowed socket of the other (such as the pelvis). In both types, bone is in indirect contact with bone through a protective layer of cartilage on the end of each, which cushions against friction and helps prevent wear and tear, and, of course, pain. Between the cartilaginous ends of the bones is a sac containing synovial fluid, which is vital to keep the joint lubricated.

The bones of your back – the vertebrae – are also jointed, and separated with discs of cartilage which help to keep the joints stable.

Tendons and ligaments are the connecting fibres which join muscle to bone. They are made up of elastic lengths of tissue called collagen, which criss-cross over each other and which can stretch and contract again millions and millions of times.

Muscles are made up of millions of fibres which can store and release energy. There are two different types of muscle fibres – 'slow acting' fibres and 'fast acting' ones – and they work in different ways. Slow acting fibres enable us to withstand comparatively prolonged exercise; fast ones contract twice as fast as the slow types, which means they respond to tasks (or exercise) requiring quick, strong action. Most people have both types in their body in more or less equal proportions, but the sort of life you lead, the work you do and the exercise you undertake can change these proportions. People who need to use their energy in short bursts, for extremely heavy lifting, for example, or for running short distances very fast, will look bulky and 'muscular' because of their higher proportion of 'fast' fibres.

People whose work or exercise demands a high level of endurance over longer periods of time will have proportionately more slow acting fibres in their muscles and will look a lot leaner. Think about the difference between the body of a champion 100m runner, for example, and the runners who tend to be among the first finishers in marathons.

What Might Start Going Wrong?

For many people, there is a gradual but fairly relentless loss in suppleness as they get older. It may become harder, and even more painful, to reach up that last inch or two when getting a suitcase from the top of the wardrobe, or prolonged walking may produce aches and pains in the back or the legs. We may get twinges and tweaks in our shoulders, neck and knees. Unhappily, about 80 per cent of the over-50s show some joint deterioration to a greater or lesser degree.

You can strain a ligament by pushing it beyond its natural capacity to contract back. This is more likely to happen if you are unused to vigorous exercise and go hell for leather one day, or if you exercise without warming up first.

A process inevitable with age is the thinning of bones, known as osteoporosis, and some people are unfortunate enough to suffer very badly, with a great deal of pain as the bones actually shrink in size. This can cause loss of height, twisting and deformity of the skeleton, and great discomfort as the internal organs may be displaced by the pressure of the changing skeleton. In the worst cases, the loss of mobility can be very serious. Osteoporosis also predisposes to fractures, which in themselves are painful and disabling.

Also, muscles can literally waste away through lack of use, and it's this lack of use, rather than the effect of ageing itself, that prevents our muscles retaining their capacity to store and release energy and to keep us supple, strong and mobile. If you are ever ill and forced to become immobile, you'll see the effects of muscle-wasting in a relatively short time, even days. The phrase 'use it or lose it' leaps to mind!

One of the commonest causes of lack of mobility is back pain – at some point, it's estimated, 80 per cent of us will suffer from some sort of disabling lower back pain. More working days are lost through this in the UK than for any other reason. After heart disease, it's the most common disabling condition and while it can affect all ages, your chances of contracting it increase as you get older. The causes of back pain are still baffling the experts, and drastic 'cures' which involve surgery may only help about 1 per cent of sufferers, and could even make some conditions worse. Nevertheless, it does seem as though many cases are caused, or made worse, by poor posture, which can often be corrected.

Do You Have to Lose Suppleness as You Get Older?

Some of this chapter's already starting to sound depressing but deterioration is by no means unavoidable, as so many active, fit and supple older people already know. There are changes you can make to your life that will help you to maintain mobility. And you can make these changes at any age, though the sooner the better!

You can stay supple by paying attention to your diet and to your lifestyle. Many older people, and their doctors, can testify how effective these changes are.

Diet and Exercise

Before you start making changes to your lifestyle, though, it's wise to check with your doctor. This is especially true if you have any joint and muscle pain or weakness and back pain – these always need proper investigation by your doctor.

If you do need treatment for an underlying condition, some treatments can have unpleasant and unwanted effects.

Once you have sought medical advice for any problems, you can start to put into practice your new programme. In the next couple of chapters and in the next section of this book, we'll look at changes and additions you can make to your diet. You'll also find some special exercises to help you stay supple.

Chapter Five

Every Day, in Every Way, You're Lightening Up!

As we've seen, a certain amount of stiffening up has been accepted as part of getting older, and we lose our general elasticity as tissues thicken and dry all the way through our body – just as on the outside our skin appears more lined and less 'springy' to the touch, so too our internal tissues can lose their 'bounce'.

We can, though, do a great deal to keep flexible and maintain our body's ability to stretch and move freely.

Start by standing, and sitting, right!

All of us get into bad habits in our daily actions and it can become more natural to slouch than to stand and sit correctly. But this does our circulation no favours at all and puts extra unnecessary strain on all parts of the skeleton. Continually bad posture can also contribute to back ache.

It's so easy to forget how much more energetic we look and feel when standing straight, with proper attention to posture – and how easy it is to ignore the fact that a slumped outline makes us look, and even feel, older than we need be!

The correct way to stand may feel as if it resists everything that's 'normal' to you, but with practice, it does stop feeling odd. You can maintain the right posture whether you're standing or sitting, walking or exercising, and in time it will become second nature. It will improve your co-ordination and your control of your body, and allow you to 'hold' the body in a more physiological way – the way it was meant to be.

Here's what to do:

- Think about where your head is and resist the 'natural' tendency to bend it forwards or downwards. Gently raise your chin and be aware of your head 'sitting' or 'balancing' on your spine.
- Tense and then relax your shoulders, and then 'unround' them gently. Make sure you don't tense them again in an exaggerated 'soldierly' way.
- Breathe in and out regularly and fairly slowly.
- Tilt your pelvis very slightly forward by tucking in your bottom.
- Contract your abdominal muscles by holding in your tummy.
- Keep your feet and knees slightly apart.

Feel how your weight becomes evenly distributed, and how your head, shoulders and hips aren't tilted one way or the other. Your spine is now in alignment, without any curves or kinks that aren't meant to be there.

To avoid tension or strain:

- Keep breathing.
- Keep your mouth slightly open, without clenched teeth or pursed lips.
- Don't shove your tongue into the roof of your mouth – keep it loose!

Keep checking your posture when standing or sitting. Don't sit for long in the same position. If you're at the theatre or the cinema, try and get up every 30–60 minutes and avoid slumping.

Deskbound?

Do you sit at a desk for much of your day? Watch out! Persistent stiffness, back ache and repetitive strain injury (RSI) are all caused by poor posture.

Here are some basic safety features to help promote and retain good posture and flexibility:

- Check your desk and seat height – you should be able to use a keyboard comfortably, without needing to place your arms in a 'sit up and beg' pose.

- Never sit with your legs crossed! Instead, place them flat on the floor. If you're small and your chair can't be lowered to make this possible, use a foot rest.

- Keep your back straight and supported, and don't be tempted to sit forward.

- Avoid RSI by taking a rest from typing every half hour or more for a minute or two. RSI is a painful condition, caused by joint inflammation, that prevents you using your hands and fingers. Tingling pains or numbness are early warning signs. If you have an attack, the only real cure is to rest your hands, sometimes for weeks.

Yoga for Mobility

One of the best ways of learning about stretching and suppleness is through yoga.

Yoga 'opens out' the skeleton to prevent us from locking ourselves into the same actions, the same movements, that place wear and tear on joints and muscles. It allows the body to learn new ways of moving and, in doing so, loosens up all the tissue of the body.

Devotees of yoga say it not only challenges the body, but also clears the mind, and it can be a wonderful stress-beater. It's suitable for all ages and all levels of fitness and suppleness.

You can learn yoga from a book – there are some good ones available, which clearly illustrate the stretches and exercises. But beginners are best with a teacher, either one to one or in a class. You progress at your own rate and it's especially important to have instruction if you already have specific joint problems or any other condition that's restricting your normal everyday movement.

There are different forms of yoga, some with a greater spiritual content than others, though most people going to classes in the UK are more interested in the physical, revitalising benefits, rather than the philosophy behind it all. None of the forms are especially 'easy', though, and at times holding a stretch can be very difficult indeed!

For people who like brisk, fast-paced exercise, yoga may feel a bit tame and slow. It may not be for you. But those who decide to stay with yoga often maintain it's a way of life for them, a necessary and pleasurable activity that they miss if they can't do it.

Angela Rippon and Yoga

Angela has been practising yoga for about five years now. 'I can't remember why I took it up – it just appealed to me because I felt it would be relaxing and a good way to keep supple.'

She now reckons she's at a 'medium to advanced' level. 'Week by week, you can feel yourself becoming better at it, as you work your body that little bit harder.' Some of the stretches she has learnt are now part of her regular early morning 'wake up' routine.

Angela does a class most weeks. 'It lasts one to one and half hours, and there are anything between six and 20 of us there. There are both sexes and all ages. The great thing about yoga is that you don't have to be as "good" as the person beside you in the class – you do what you can do and make progress as quickly as *you* want to.'

Angela likes the physical effect of regular yoga. 'It keeps the body flexible and trim, and it makes you think what your body can do. It makes you feel good, basically – I know it's reckoned to be very beneficial for the internal organs as well as the muscles. There's a psychological benefit, as well. You concentrate on your body for that time in the class and you can empty your mind of everything else, so it's wonderfully relaxing.'

Daily Stretching

Our fit-in-a-month exercise plan incorporates stretching and flexibility exercises, but a daily programme of specific stretching is a great habit to get into.

You don't need to set aside a great chunk of time for

this – it's frequency, not intensity or length, that's the key factor in bringing you the benefits of regular stretching. Ten minutes a day is fine, and if you can only manage five, that's better than nothing!

The important thing is to keep it up. If you aim to build stretching into your routine, just as you do with other sorts of personal care like brushing your teeth or combing your hair, you'll find you can stick at it better.

Many people find the best time to stretch is on getting up in the morning, and of course, the easy thing about this form of exercise is that you can literally do it anywhere, without any special equipment or clothing. However, make sure you have enough space and a warm room with a soft surface you can lie on. Stretch in loose clothing (night clothes or underwear are fine and will save you changing into something else) and in bare feet or trainers.

With daily practice, it won't take more than a couple of weeks for you to notice some improvement in your suppleness. The benefits will increase the longer you do it.

Here are our suggested key stretches. You should be able to manage all of them, unless you have a specific joint or mobility problem. Repeat each exercise between 5 and 15 times, depending on time available and your level of flexibility.

1. *To work the chest and upper body:* Stand with arms raised above the head, fingers pointing upwards, thumbs touching each other. Straighten the elbows without 'locking' them. Move your arms back so your ears are in front of them. Now, lean backwards slowly and gently, feeling the stretch on your back.
2. *To work the tummy:* Kneel, keeping your head up and

your back straight and holding your tummy in. Now place your hands on your hips. Gently lean backwards as far as is comfortable. Feeling the stretch across your tummy and shoulders is good. As you become more flexible you will be able to lean further.

3. *To work your lower back:* Lie on the floor and bend your legs, keeping your knees together and your feet flat on the floor. Now move your knees to the right and push them as far as you can. Repeat, pushing them to the left.

4. *To work your lower back once more:* Stay in the position you're in at the beginning of exercise three, with your knees together once more. Push your lower back into the floor, by tilting your pelvis slightly. Now raise your back, lifting your bottom off the floor. Lower gently.

5. *To work the backs of your thighs:* Stay on the floor and sit up with your legs stretched out in front of you and your feet together. Lean forward with your head between your upper arms and your arms stretched out. Try to touch your toes. You'll get nearer as you improve!

Note: Check your posture at all times *(see page 48).*

Weight-Bearing for Bone Health

Osteoporosis *(see page 43)* can be alleviated, and even prevented, by regular exercise. To be more effective, this should include some weight-bearing. This might be through jogging, running, walking, dancing, rowing (indoors or out) or weight-training. Research has shown that this form of exercise actually increases bone density.

To add weight, you can buy hand weights and leg weights (which strap on your ankles). A can of beans in each hand or a bag of rice strapped on each ankle will do the job just as well. Many of the stretches and movements described in this book can be done with hand and/or leg weights. Start off with a small weight (100–200g) and work up to weights of a kilogram each.

Alexander Technique

This technique, sometimes known as 'the Alexander principle', is a form of postural therapy originally devised in the twentieth century by Australian F. M. Alexander. It aims to recondition the way you move, stand and use your limbs in order to prevent and correct what teachers of the technique would regard as constant misuse. The therapy claims successes in curing or improving a wide range of disorders, including osteoarthritis, high blood pressure, back pain, chronic fatigue and others, using movements a teacher can train you to do and which you can then practise at home. The movements are devised individually for you, and will make you feel more supple and generally more toned and relaxed.

If you feel this technique would help you, see a qualified therapist. Most offer one-to-one therapy, though there are also classes in some parts of the country.

The Pilates Method

Pilates – pronounced *Pi-lar-tis*, which is the name of its founder – is a system of movements, stretches and exercises that shape the body, counter the effects of poor posture, and help repair and restore damage to the skeleton and the muscles. It's a method of achieving fitness and suppleness by body conditioning, and it became highly fashionable in the 1980s, when several famous actors, dancers and athletes discovered it.

From the East

Here are some therapies from the East:

- Shiatsu, a form of therapeutic massage from Japan, is rather like acupuncture without the needles. It uses pressure, massage and exercise to treat the whole body, or specific parts of it. Therapists offer a single session, or a series of sessions, depending on what they suggest might help. It's essentially a form of relaxation as well as a means of relieving pain, and you can learn simple exercises to do at home. It claims success with a range of muscular and joint disorders. Some therapists now teach a shiatsu that involves 'dynamic stretching', incorporating shiatsu principles into a whole-body series of exercises.
- *T'ai Chi* – Sometimes described as 'meditation in motion', T'ai Chi is a Chinese movement therapy which looks like a graceful, tranquil dance. Widely practised in China, it's becoming more and more popular in the West. Its devotees say it is a relaxing body and mind toner, which brings benefits without strain or stress.
- *Aikido* – This ancient martial art from Japan is a spiritual as well as a physical discipline, and not necessarily seen as a therapy. However, teachers of Aikido say their pupils find their joints are freer, their circulation is improved and suppleness is greatly increased.

The Pilates method is ideally tailored to the individual, and its trained teachers sometimes work one to one to devise a programme that fits you exactly. People who have benefited from the Pilates method include sufferers of osteoporosis and severe back pain, those new to exercise and people wanting to combine exercise with relieving stress.

Get De-Stressed!

Pressures from work or other areas of your life can cause stress and tension – and both of these may affect you physically. Everyone needs time off in order to function better in every way.

Angela Rippon has a hectic working schedule, but she's careful to build relaxation time into it. 'I've learnt over the years that I need to plan for "me time", time I can take away from London or work – it doesn't just happen,' she says. 'If I see from my diary that I have an especially busy and pressured number of weeks ahead, I make sure I can plan a long weekend away from it in the middle.'

As a routine treat, Angela finds having a massage is a great restorative. 'I love going to the cinema with friends, too,' she adds, 'but a favourite way to switch off is really simple – I read a book.'

You can find addresses for information on what you might do to relax and ideas for further reading on page 127.

Chapter Six
The Fats of Life – the Role of Fish Oils

The health role of certain oils has been known for centuries, but it's only in the last 20 to 30 years that scientific research has fully demonstrated how valuable they can be.

The message we tend to receive from the media these days is that fats and oils are bad for us. This just isn't true – or, rather, it's misleading. Some fats are essential to health and, indeed, life itself. Some are known as 'essential fatty acids', or EFAs, because we cannot manufacture them in the body and they have to be obtained in the diet.

It is important to ensure that our diet includes enough of these important nutrients to stay healthy. In particular, Omega 6 and Omega 3 EFAs (the names are derived from their chemical structure). Many people's diets are high in the sort of fats which actually prevent the body from making good use of the few EFAs they do take in.

Omega 3 fats have a vital health role. They help maintain a healthy heart and circulation and keep joints supple and flexible. The body uses Omega 3 fats to manufacture prostaglandins, chemicals which regulate the activity of cells in every part of the body.

Omega 3 fats are found naturally in fish and marine vegetables ('seaweeds'), in some seeds and in some nuts. Populations which naturally eat a lot of fish, such as the Japanese and the Eskimos (who also eat seal meat, getting a secondary benefit from the fish-only diet of the seal), are less likely to go short of Omega 3 fats; vegans, who eat more seeds and nuts than others, have a higher level of Omega 3 in their body fat than most 'average' Westerners.

Cod Liver Oil

Cod liver oil is a rich source of Omega 3 (and other important nutrients, which we'll look at later). Here we'll look at how it may help maintain the function of your joints.

Cod liver oil has been commercially available for generations. Fishermen would remove the livers of their cod catch at sea and toss them into a bucket to ferment for weeks. The resulting oil was then sold to the tanning industry and to farmers as animal feed.

At first cod liver oil's health benefits were attributed to its vitamin content (it is a rich source of vitamins A and D) but subsequent research discovered that it was an excellent source of the valuable Omega 3 oils.

Since the 1950s, more and more people have taken cod liver oil to keep their joints supple and flexible.

Since then cod liver oil's popularity has grown and today it is the single most popular health supplement in Britain.

Your Dietary Changes

A good, wholesome diet based on a variety of foods is the best recipe for health and is a good way of helping maintain joint mobility. Eating well helps fuel the body's own resources and both doctors and the Department of Health recognise the importance of a diet high in oily fish. Although more information on healthy eating is covered in the next chapter, the Family Health Authority suggest eating two or three fish meals a week in order to supply Omega 3 fatty acids.

The oily fish widely available in this country include mackerel, herring and sardines but today many people find it more convenient and palatable to take a daily measure of cod liver oil in capsule form. Care should be taken when purchasing cod liver oil capsules, as not all contain the same percentage of the valuable Omega 3s which help to maintain the suppleness in the joints.

Chapter Seven

Exercise for Everyone!

Improve your Fitness – in Just One Month!

Here's a programme you really can begin from a standing start. Whatever your previous experience of exercise, or your current state of activity, this step-by-step programme is safe, effective and enjoyable – and the great thing is you'll see, and feel, results in just four weeks. It's not time-consuming, either. By the end of week four, you'll be cramming a worthwhile session into just 35 minutes at a time.

Remember, exercise is best done regularly. Shortish periods of exercise several times a week will do you more good than a fortnight's inactivity punctuated by a single exhausting afternoon. Aim to get to the stage where you miss exercising if you're prevented from doing it for more than a few days. If it helps to fix a time and a day, mark it in your diary.

Research shows that getting the motivation up to start exercising is relatively easy. It's sticking at it where so many of us fail. Read our tips on beating the boredom fact (see page 86) if you need a motivational boost.

Our programme combines the three forms of exercise you should include to ensure all-round fitness and suppleness:

1. Energy-boosting aerobic exercise, which improves the functioning of your heart by raising your heart rate and giving it just that little bit more work to do. Regular aerobic exercise (also called 'cardio-vascular exercise' because of the way it targets the heart and the circulation) increases your stamina. In time, you'll find you can do more of any activity without feeling tired. It also improves the functioning of your other organs, including your lungs and your digestive system. Weight-bearing exercise (any exercise involving walking or running) is also excellent for building bone strength; this form of exercise can be an important factor in both the treatment and prevention of osteoporosis.
2. Mobility-boosting exercises which target your joints. Activities involving stretching, lifting or bending will then become easier.
3. Strengthening exercises for your muscles, which will not only allow you to do more intensive, energetic activities, but will also improve your appearance – let's face it, well-toned muscle looks a lot better than flab – and your posture.

Note: For the best all-round exercise, your regular activity should have elements of all three forms at every session. That's the format we have here. But if you find this difficult to do for whatever reason (available time, place or preference), then it's fine to concentrate on each element on its own, perhaps focusing on one one day by spending twice or three times as long on it, then spending time on another the following day.

If you have any doubts about your health or strength, if you have never exercised before, or if you have a condition which requires medical attention, please check with your doctor before you begin this or any other exercise programme. And remember, never exercise through pain. *If it hurts, stop.*

As for clothing, you don't need special fitness gear for exercising. Anything comfortable which does not restrict your movement in any way is fine. Footwear can be trainers if you're jogging or well-fitting flat shoes if you're just walking.

Golden Rules

- *Always make sure your posture is comfortable and correct* when beginning any exercise. Standing or sitting, hold your head up, don't slump your shoulders, and have your back straight. If you're on your feet, tuck in your bottom.
- *Always warm up* before you begin any exercise session. This makes sure your muscles, ligaments and connective tissue are gently stretched in preparation, which will help prevent straining. Cold muscles are more prone to injury. It also raises your heart rate and gets your circulation working well.
- *Always cool down* at the end of your session. This helps prevent any build-up of excess fluid which could cause stiffness in your limbs – that's often the main reason behind any aches and pains people get the day following exercise.
- *Build up to fitness* over time. If you exhaust yourself, your motivation will disappear as the novelty wears off all too quickly. Becoming too tired too quickly increases the risk of strain and has little effect on fitness levels. Stick to the programme and you'll find you can do *measurably more* at the end of the four weeks before becoming fatigued.

- *Each week, aim to exercise between three and five times* over the seven days. You can do more if you wish. Moderate exercise of this type is fine every day. Professional athletes and people who exercise or train intensively usually aim for one rest day in seven. You don't need to. However, while even one session a week is better than nothing at all, you will need to complete at least three sessions to see results in a month.

Week One

The first week's sessions each last about 15 minutes. Move as swiftly as you can from each exercise to the next.

Warm Up

Warm up with these movements. To complete them should take you about three minutes.

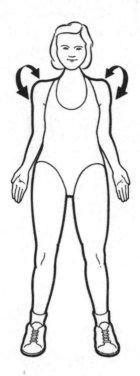

FIG 1.

Warm up your shoulders

- Stand with your feet shoulder width apart and rotate your shoulders six times to the front, then six times to the back.
- Repeat three times, slightly more vigorously each time.

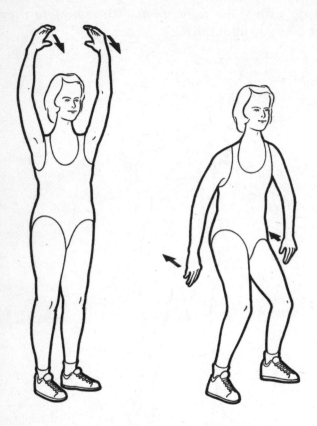

FIG 2.

Swing your arms

- Start with your arms above your head and swing them down and behind, bending your knees slightly as you do so.
- Straighten up as you bring your arms up above your head once more.
- Repeat five times.

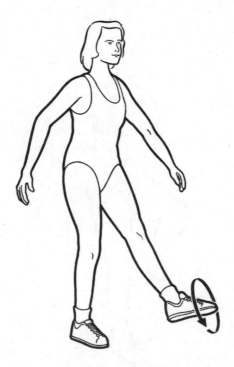

FIG. 3.

Get your legs and feet going!

- Stand up straight and raise one leg in front of you. Circle your foot six times one way, then six times the other. (Do this sitting down if you have to, or with a hand on a chair back to steady yourself.)
- Repeat with the other leg.
- Repeat three times.

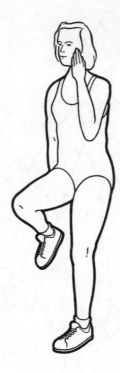

FIG. 4.

Brisk march

- March briskly up and down on the spot for 30 seconds.

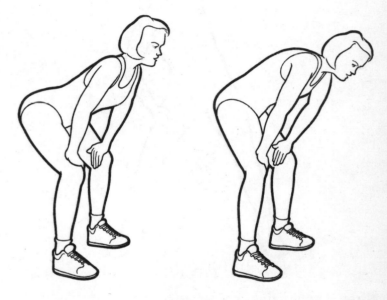

FIG. 5.

Stretch your back

- Stand with your feet apart, knees bent, hands resting on your thighs.
- Slightly bend your back, curving it outwards and pulling in your tummy. Hold for a count of two.
- Repeat three times.

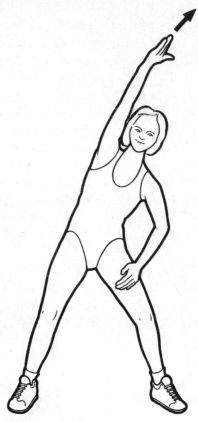

FIG. 6.

Stretch your sides

- Stand straight with your feet apart, keeping your knees slightly bent. Keeping your body straight and your head looking forward, stretch your arm upwards as far as you can and bend sideways at the waist. Hold for a count of two.
- Repeat on the other side.
- Repeat three times.

Get Moving

Once you've done your stretches, you can get moving by doing an activity you can keep up for five to six minutes without stopping for a rest. Here are some suggestions:

- Walking – round the block, round the garden or up and down the High Street if you want to. You can even go up and down stairs in your house. Keep your pace as brisk as you can.
- Jogging (but only if you can do this without getting more than a little out of breath).
- Cycling, either on a stationary exercise cycle or a 'real' one.

You can combine these activities and even insert a minute or so's skipping or fast marching on the spot.

If you're out of condition or overweight, you may feel you're moving very slowly. That's OK. Aim to reach a level of intensity which challenges you but which doesn't stop you being able to have a normal conversation. 'Slightly out of breath' is the state you should target, as this shows you've raised your heart rate and got your body *working*. Your actual speed is not so crucial. You may not be fast, but you should find you move more quickly as you get fitter.

Get Mobile, Get Strong

Now it's time to get mobile and strong with a series of movements which target your joints and your muscles, allowing you to feel more flexible and supple. Spend about four minutes on this sequence.

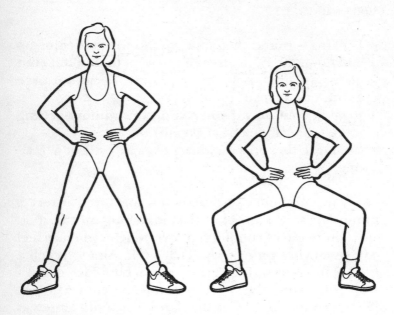

FIG. 7.

Squats

- With your feet quite wide apart, place your hands on your hips.
- Keeping your back as straight as you can, lower yourself into a squatting position then rise up again.
- Repeat five times.

(Don't worry if you can't get down very far! You'll get better with practice. If necessary, hold the back of a chair with one hand to steady yourself at first.)

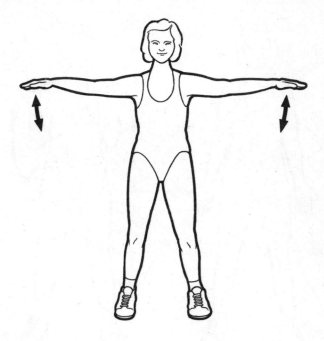

FIG. 8.

Arm raises

- Stand with your feet shoulder width apart and your arms at your sides. Raise your arms up and out slowly until they're at shoulder height. Lower equally slowly. Repeat eight times.

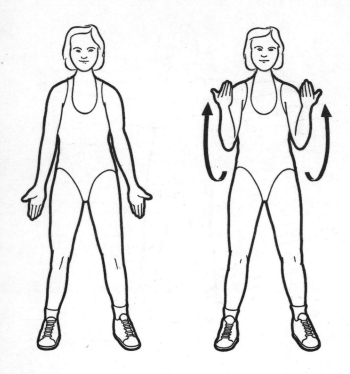

FIG. 9.

Hand raises

- Stand as before, with your arms by your sides and the palms of your hands to the front. Tuck your upper arms into your sides.
- Bend your elbows, so your hands come up to your shoulders, keeping your elbows close to your sides.
- Repeat eight times.

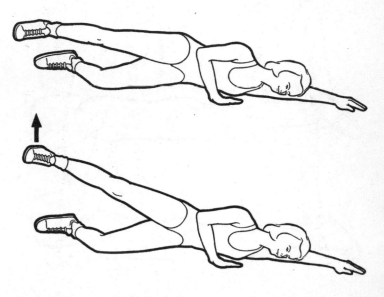

FIG. 10.

Leg lifts

- Lie on your side, with your arm outstretched and your head resting on it. Bend your lower leg.
- Raise your upper leg slowly, making sure your leg stays straight and your hips are in a straight line. Lower it equally slowly.
- Repeat six times, then turn over and do the same with the other leg.

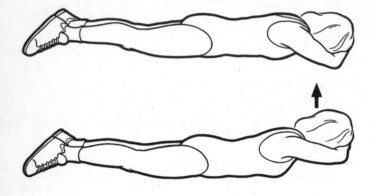

FIG. 11.

Shoulder lifts

- Lie on your tummy with your feet slightly apart. Try to press your hips into the floor. Place your head on your arms.
- Raise your head and shoulders, keeping your legs and feet on the floor. Feel the stretch in your back.
- Repeat six times.

Cool Down

Cool down for two minutes or so with these relaxing stretches.

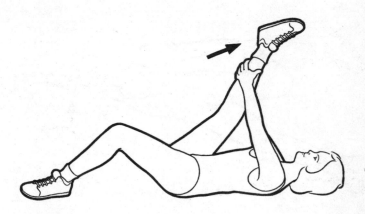

FIG. 12.

Hamstring stretch

- Lie on your back with your knees bent. Slowly bring one leg towards your chest and then stretch it out as far as you can, keeping your hands behind your calf.
- Pull your leg in and feel the stretch down your thigh. Hold for a count of five.
- Repeat with the other leg.

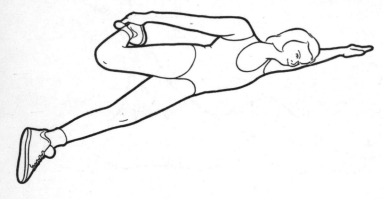

FIG. 13.

Thigh stretch

- Lie on your side with lower arm outstretched support-ing your head. Bend your upper leg and reach back with your upper arm and grasp the instep of your foot.
- Pull in your foot as far as you can, gently and slowly. Hold for a count of four and then release.
- Turn over and repeat with the other leg.

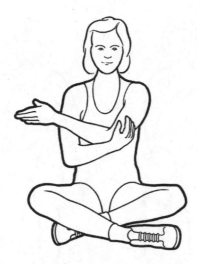

FIG. 14.

Shoulder stretch

- Sit on the floor with your back straight, cross-legged if you can. Bring your arm across your chest and with your other hand press your elbow into your chest.
- At the same time, press the shoulder of your upper arm down and really feel the stretch. Hold for a count of four and release.
- Repeat with the other arm.

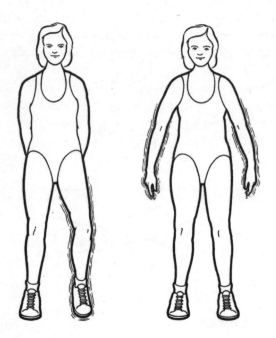

FIG. 15.

Shake out!

- Stand up and shake out your legs, and then your arms.

Week Two

On this second week, you should aim to spend about 20 minutes on each session.

Warm up as Week One.

Get moving as Week One, but this time make it last a little longer. You should manage eight to nine minutes of continuous activity by now, again avoiding exhaustion and retaining enough breath to be able to talk.

Get mobile, get strong as Week One, adding the following exercises to your routine. You can insert these extras between any of the existing exercises. This sequence should last about five minutes.

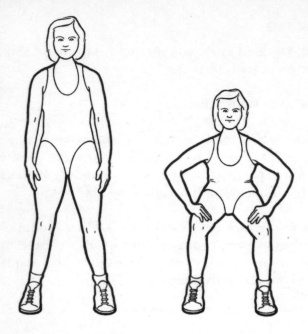

FIG. 16.

Sitting on air

- Stand straight, with your feet shoulder width apart. Bend forward with your hands on your thighs, bending at the knees, as if you were 'sitting' in mid-air. Keep your head up.
- Slowly return to the starting position.
- Repeat six times.

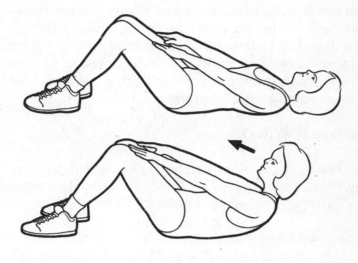

FIG. 17.

Stomach pulls

- Lie on your back with your knees bent. Press your back into the floor. Bring your hands up to your thighs.
- Pull your tummy in and tighten your pelvic floor muscles (the ones you'd use if you were trying to stem a flow of urine). At the same time, raise your shoulders up off the floor. Return slowly.
- Repeat six times.

Note: Breathe out as you rise and in as you lower yourself.

Cool down as Week One.

Week Three

By now, if you've been exercising regularly, you should already be feeling a difference in the ease with which you can do some of the stretches. Go at your own pace – but don't let that be an excuse for avoiding challenge! You should feel refreshed and relaxed at the end of each session – and if you are ever stiff the next day, concentrate on cooling down effectively. During this week, your sessions should last 25 minutes at a time.

Warm up as Week One.

Get moving in the usual way, but again, take more time, say 12 to 14 minutes, over this section. This might mean it's worthwhile doing something different:

• Try swimming – and instead of your usual warm up, shake out your legs and arms for half a minute or so at the side of the pool, and do two lengths fairly slowly. Then do as many lengths as you can in your allotted time without reaching the point of total fatigue.
   If you can't swim, walk across the shallow end and back. Feel yourself pushing against the water. Try going backwards as well as forwards. Water provides a resistance and therefore a challenge which gives a highly effective work-out.

Get mobile, get strong as Week Two, but increase the number of repetitions to 10 each time. This should take you approximately 10 minutes.

Cool down as before.

Week Four

By the end of this week, you will have built up to a routine which you can use as a way of maintaining your level of fitness for as long as you wish. Aim to complete this routine or its equivalent three to five times every week.

You may find you need to increase the intensity of your routine in order to keep up its effect. You can do this in a number of ways:

- Increase the number of repetitions you do – the last one or two of every set should be difficult (though not almost impossible or painful). If exercise is *too* easy, it's not doing you any good!
- Use hand weights during your exercise sequences. You can buy special ones at sports shops, but a couple of large baked bean cans are just as good. This makes sure you're really working your muscles and giving yourself a little more resistance.
- Ensure your aerobic exercise is more demanding by running instead of walking, swimming faster than you're used to, carrying a backpack during your walks or cycling faster.

Warm up as before, but increase it by one or two minutes.

Get moving as before, but again increasing your time so you are spending 20 minutes in continuous energetic movement. You may vary the speed or intensity, but don't slow down to a stop!

Get mobile, get strong as Week Three, increasing the repetitions to 12 at a time. You'll be doing the whole sequence more quickly than before, so it may take you slightly less time than before, say about eight or nine minutes.

Cool down as Week Three.

Keep It Up!

Don't let exercise become a chore – you'll soon give it up if you can't look forward to it. Here are some ideas on making it more fun:

- Exercise with a friend – you're less likely to drop out if it means letting someone down.
- Exercise out of doors when you can – try doing your routine in the park (if you're with someone else you'll soon get over feeling self-conscious about it!)
- Join a class – they're everywhere *(see page 00)*.
- Form your own class with friends. Exercise in your own sitting room to different videos (borrowed from the library or hired from the video shop). Ring the changes.
- Use a personal radio/stereo during your routine.
- Join a gym where you can watch TV while you exercise.
- Get up extra early and get your exercise done for the day – you'll really feel set up and pleased with yourself!
- Read while you 'work' – a magazine or a book can be propped up on the exercise cycle at home or in the gym.
- Exercise to music – though be careful not to make it *too* slow or serene!

Well done! If you've come this far and stuck to the programme, you should now:

- feel generally fitter and more energetic
- feel firmer, especially on your arms and legs
- experience less breathlessness when doing anything demanding strength and energy
- feel proud of yourself!

Section Three

STAY HEALTHY

Introduction

This section deals with something of interest to everyone – food and eating it!

Here we look at how your daily diet affects your health and how you can change things for the better. Our eating plan focuses on a whole range of healthy dishes that offer you new ideas over a fortnight, plus a selection of recipes for meals that may be new to you. You may already be eating well, if so, well done! But you'll still find at least a couple of ideas here to add variety.

We also talk here about the role of dietary supplements. I take ginseng, evening primrose oil and cod liver oil every day, and I certainly feel they maintain my health and energy levels. There are a number of times in our life when we may go short of everything we need: we may be stressed, extra busy, recovering after illness, or just getting older. Maybe supplements could help you. We'll explain more on pages 106-8.

Angela Rippon

Chapter Eight

Healthy Eating: The Basics

If you read newspapers and magazines, or watch TV, you'll be aware that anything to do with eating, food and nutrition is perennially hot news. The latest food scares vie for space with information and advice on healthy eating. Cookery programmes include information on whether the dishes they demonstrate are 'healthy', while health programmes routinely investigate diet. If you're aware of any of this, you'll realise it's now well known that there is a link between good health and nutrition, and your choice of food could have a long-term effect on your well-being.

Yet despite the messages coming at us from all sides, we're still following the trend set in America for health-threatening obesity. Too many people are still eating poor quality diets high in saturated fat and sugar, which may increase our risk of illness.

The advice on healthy eating doesn't seem to make as much impact on us as the habits we've grown up with – and yet we have changed. For instance, how many of us ate yoghurt when we were children? Probably the only spaghetti most of us ate before the seventies tended to come out of a tin. A meal wasn't a meal if it didn't have a centrepiece of meat and if it wasn't followed by a nice big plateful of stodgy pud!

We have broadened our tastebuds in the last 20 to 30 years – so the next step should be to make further changes to our eating habits in order to change the proportions of different nutrients, giving us a healthier balance.

Healthy eating shouldn't be difficult to achieve, especially as there is now widespread agreement among nutritionists about the principles of a healthy diet. The healthy diet is low in *fat*, high in *carbohydrate*, contains plenty of *vitamins and minerals*, enough *protein*, and is high in *fibre*. Yes, controversy still rages about the details, and research is still going on to measure the impact of diet on aspects of health. We still have much to learn about why some people are more susceptible to the ill-effects of poor diet than others, and how great its relative importance is to other factors, including your genetic inheritance, the amount you exercise and whether or not you smoke or have ever smoked. Nevertheless, while the debate goes on, there are guidelines you can follow with confidence:

• Major overhauls to your diet which involve drastic cutbacks or punishing regimes don't work! You're more likely to stick with smaller, gradual changes. Frankly, highly restricted diets which mean you go without certain groups of foods can even be harmful, unless you follow them under professional supervision.

• Stick to two or three moderately sized meals each day, rather than semi-starving yourself for much of the day and having one mega-sized meal to compensate. Your digestive system works better on a regular supply of food.

- Snacking between meals is fine, but make sure you don't always choose crisps, cakes or chocolate, which are high in sugars and/or fats. A piece of fruit or a raw vegetable provides proportionately more vitamins, minerals and fibre.
- Increase your intake of unrefined cereals (wholemeal bread, pasta and rice).
- Reduce your intake of saturated fats (the fats mainly found in animal-origin products).
- Aim to eat five portions of fruit and vegetables each day.

Low in Fat...

All human beings need fats in their daily diet. The two kinds of fat we eat are known as *saturated* – found in meats and animal products such as eggs, milk and cheese – and *unsaturated* – in seeds, nuts and fish. In addition, unsaturated fats are divided into two groups, *monounsaturated* (in olive oil, for example) and *polyunsaturated* (in nuts and seeds).

Essential polyunsaturated fats have been discussed on page 57. They cannot be manufactured by the body and must be obtained from the diet. These polyunsaturated fats provide us with Omega 6 and Omega 3 oils – both vital to health *(see pages 57–59)*.

Saturated fats are not an essential part of the diet and all the nutrients they contain can be found in other foods. However, that's not to say the healthy diet contains no saturated fat. It's the amount, or rather the proportion, of saturated fat that can be the problem. Too much, and there is a risk of obesity and disease.

According to the Institute for Optimum Nutrition, the ideal diet has 20 per cent of its overall calories as fat. Of this, a third should be saturated, a third polyunsaturated and a third monounsaturated. In particular, we should take care to maintain or improve our intake of Omega 6 and Omega 3 fats. The body must get Omega 3 direct from the diet, as it can't synthesise it from anything else, but Omega 3 fats are especially likely to be in short supply in the modern diet as a result of increasing reliance on processed foods and the popularity of Omega 6 based oils and margarines.

High in Carbohydrate...

Carbohydrate fuels the body. It is found in all grains and cereals, pulses, sugars, vegetables and fruits. Some carbohydrates are 'slow release', because they contain more complex carbohydrate and sometimes more fibre. The body needs to break this down and convert it into glucose in the liver. Others are 'fast release', as the glucose is already there in the food.

Sweet foods – honey, sugar – are quick release; starchy foods – pasta, potatoes, cereals, pulses – are slow release. Some foods have sugar and starch in them. Foods which are either slow release or a combination of sugar and starch (such as fruits) give better 'food value' than the 'quick fix' energy buzz of a chocolate bar, which leaves you feeling hungry shortly afterwards when the glucose 'high' drops, rapidly lowering the blood sugar level. Refined carbohydrates – white flour, white rice, white bread – are lower in nutrients than their unrefined counterparts, as the refining process removes some to their vitamins and minerals. People who have glucose-related health problems need to take care with their intake of fast-release carbohydrates.

In a healthy diet, carbohydrate makes up 55 to 70 per cent of our daily calorie intake.

Enough Protein...

Protein is made up of amino acids, the 'building blocks' of cells and tissue. It assists in the growth and repair and replacement of bones, muscles, connective tissues and organ walls. Protein is also used to make hormones, enzymes and antibodies.

Protein is supplied by animal-origin foods and plant-origin foods. We get it from meat, fish, milk, cheese, potatoes, pasta, grains, cereals, beans, nuts, soya and soya products.

We probably eat twice as much protein as we really need, because of its easy availability. It's difficult, in fact, to go short of protein as a normal adult unless you are on a very inadequate diet, but it's probably possible to eat too much protein. In fact, there are nutritionists who feel we routinely 'overdose' on protein. Some people with digestive problems can certainly overload their liver and kidneys if they have too much protein. The longest living peoples in the world, according to a review of the available studies in Leslie Kenton's *The New Ageless Ageing*, both today and throughout history, have survived on a diet rich in fresh, raw foods which is relatively low in energy (calories) and low in protein. However, protein foods from animal sources tend to be high in saturated fats and this in itself can present a health risk if too much is eaten.

Meat protein is considered to be 'complete' protein because it contains all the amino acids. Yet if you don't eat meat, you can get all the amino acids from non meat sources, as long as you eat a number of different plant proteins. For example, eating nuts and rice, or lentils and pasta, will give you the full complement of amino acids.

A healthy diet gets between 10 and 15 per cent of its calories from protein.

High in Fibre...

The fibre in your diet has no actual nutritional value and it has no value as a source of energy. Yet it's an important part of your daily intake. It isn't actually absorbed by the digestive system as it passes through. Instead, it keeps your system working well, because of its structure.

Fibre comes from the outer husks of grains and the skins and flesh of fruit and vegetables. The molecules which make up fibre can't be broken down by digestive juices. As a result, fibre remains intact, bulking out the faeces and drawing in water from the surrounding blood vessels of the intestine. This helps prevent constipation by ensuring the stools remain soft and easy to pass, and encourages the lower bowel to function regularly. This also means waste products don't remain in the body for long.

Increasing Fibre

It's usually better to increase the fibre content of your diet gradually and to avoid concentrated fibre sources such as unprocessed bran unless you're advised differently by your doctor. You may suffer from painful wind or abdominal cramps otherwise.

Fresh fruit and vegetables, dried fruits, wholegrain cereals and fruit and vegetable skins are good sources of fibre. Raw foods have more fibre than cooked ones.

Plenty of Vitamins...

Vitamins are micronutrients, which are needed for just about every bodily process. About 12 are known to be vital to health and nutrition. The body can make some vitamins (for example, it can synthesise vitamin D from sunlight), but the vast majority need to come from the food we eat.

Vitamins spark off the biological process of metabolism – the way the body uses food. They also have an important role to play in the repair and maintenance of the body's tissue. In particular, the antioxidant vitamins A, C and E, help protect the body's tissues against the damaging effects of free radicals and can maintain a healthy immune system.

There are disagreements about the 'RNI' of vitamins – that's the 'reference nutrient intake', formerly known as the RDA or recommended daily allowance. Some experts feel that published RNIs err on the low side and that we could benefit from higher levels of some vitamins. They also point out that individual needs may differ according to age, health, stress and so on.

However, if you can rely on having a good, healthy diet based on a variety of mainly fresh foods, you are probably getting the vitamins you need. Fruit and vegetables are an excellent source of vitamins, though be aware that cooking destroys some vitamins, as so many of them dissolve in water (which you may discard after cooking) or are affected by heat. If you often skip meals, eat poor quality food, eat a limited range of foods, have had a poor appetite due to illness or have been trying to slim, you could be going short and may benefit from a supplement *(see pages 106–9)*.

...And Minerals

There are about 6 minerals that are important for us and, like vitamins, they are vital for health. Literally thousands of functions are performed by minerals every day. For example, calcium, magnesium and phosphorus build bone, iron carries oxygen in the blood, and zinc has antioxidant functions and helps maintain the immune system.

Food Allergies

Some of us are unable to eat certain foods without an adverse reaction. This could be due to i) allergy, which means the symptoms that arise are mainly due to a response from the immune system, or ii) sensitivity or intolerance, which are rather broader terms, and less specific, as they indicate it's not known why the reaction has happened.

It's possible that some people suffer from 'leaky gut' syndrome, where undigested food particles 'escape' through the gut walls and trigger a reaction as the body meets substances it is only able to deal with in a digested, chemically deconstructed form.

It may also be that some people's immune system is more sensitive to encounters with substances that shouldn't be there. There may even be something amiss in their digestive system that prevents the metabolism of certain foods – an absent or inadequate digestive enzyme, for example.

Symptoms associated with food allergies include:

- headache, migraine
- chronic fatigue

- swelling due to fluid retention
- abdominal pain
- wind
- bowel problems
- mouth ulcers
- nausea
- joint pain
- rheumatoid arthritis
- hayfever
- persistent runny nose
- asthma
- itchy eyes
- skin rashes

All of the above symptoms may, however, have no connection with food allergy or intolerance. Always see your doctor if you have persistent symptoms. If it's suspected that your reactions are food related, seek professional help in adjusting your diet.

Some specialists in allergy testing recommend an elimination diet to isolate the offending food item. This involves having a very simple diet which consists of foods which are known to be unlikely culprits. After several days, the suspected foods are reintroduced into the diet one by one, and reactions are checked. This is actually quite difficult to do without proper support and monitoring, and continuing on an elimination diet for longer than necessary could leave you short of nutrients.

If you do suspect which food is causing you problems, cut it out of your diet for a fortnight and then introduce it once more and see if your symptoms return.

Common foods to which many people are sensitive include wheat and dairy produce, alcohol, coffee, chocolate, nuts, eggs and oranges.

Angela's Allergies

Angela Rippon discovered some years ago she couldn't eat food containing gluten (the protein found in wheat) or dairy products because of an intolerance to lactose, the sugar constituent of milk. A dietitian narrowed down Angela's diet with an exclusion diet until the guilty parties were tracked down.

'Now I avoid milk and other dairy products like the plague, as I get headaches and stomach pains if I go near them,' she says. She does, however, eat products made from soya milk, or goat's or sheep's milk, which don't contain the lactose. 'I can't eat bread or anything with gluten in it, though I occasionally allow myself a small piece of crusty French bread.' The other thing she steers clear of is red wine, and she only ever drinks small amounts of alcohol. 'I do like a glass of champagne, though,' she says. 'I think it does me good!'

Note: Health stores sell many products for people who prefer to avoid certain foods because of taste, allergy or ethics. You can buy goat's milk, for example, which has the additional benefit, like soya milk, of being lower in fat than dairy milk. Lactose-reduced cow's milk is also available. This is often acceptable to people diagnosed as lactose intolerant as the small amounts remaining in the milk may not cause a reaction. It has all the taste of cow's milk – something that substitute milks can't have, and which many people say they miss when they try other types of milk.

Chapter Nine

Food, your Health and Getting Older

The research into diet, health and ageing is fascinating, and as it increases, it becomes more and more certain that what you put on your plate makes a real difference to your chances of a healthy and lengthy middle to old age.

The main diseases to which many of us succumb in old age, those which at best slow us down and at worst end in death, are stroke, heart disease and cancer. There is excellent evidence that good nutrition reduces the chances of getting these illnesses; in addition, eating well promotes well-being and reduces the incidence and impact of less serious illness by maintaining the strength and effectiveness of the immune system.

Heart disease kills 500 people every day in the UK and is the biggest cause of premature death in both men and women. Some people are at greater risk than others of developing heart disease. These include:

- smokers
- people with high cholesterol levels (cholesterol is a fat-like substance that can clog the blood and circulatory system)
- people with high blood pressure

- people who are overweight
- people with a family history of heart disease

However, you can protect yourself and lower your risk by taking sensible measures:

- giving up smoking
- maintaining a healthy weight
- taking regular exercise and being generally physically active
- making changes to your diet

Dietary changes affect two of the main risk factors of heart disease – cholesterol levels and high blood pressure. Reducing your intake of saturated fats can lower your cholesterol level.

The Family Heart Association makes several recommendations for dietary change:

- Choose the lower fat varieties of dairy products.
- Trim visible fat from meat.
- Use spreads (butter, margarine) sparingly.
- Keep cakes, pies, pastry, biscuits and confectionery to a minimum.
- Choose foods with monounsaturated or polyunsaturated fats such as vegetables, fish, nuts and seeds.
- Cook or season with sunflower oil or olive oil.

The Department of Health recommends a minimum of two fish meals a week, one of which should be oily, as they contain the Omega 3 essential fatty acids, not saturated fats.

How do Omega 3's work? They help keep the blood flowing through the veins and arteries and minimise the risk of a blood clot.

Which Fish is Best?

For a nation surrounded by sea, we don't eat a lot of fish. Many of us prefer meat, though fish is actually easier and quicker to prepare. The best fish for essential fatty acids, including Omega 3, are the so-called 'oily fish'. Here's a list of them:

- anchovies
- bass
- carp
- crab
- halibut
- herring
- lake trout
- mackerel
- mullet
- oysters
- pilchards
- rainbow trout
- red snapper
- salmon
- sardines
- shrimp
- sole
- sprats
- squid
- swordfish
- tuna

Fresh tuna is better than canned, but if you use canned, choose the sort in brine rather than vegetable oil.

Very fresh fish can be eaten raw for maximum nutritional benefit, as the Japanese do, but it's hard to be sure any fish you buy is fresh enough for this. When cooking fish, baking, boiling, steaming or grilling fish preserves the essential fatty acids better than frying.

Weight Control and Fat

The body's capacity for storing carbohydrate and protein is limited, and it metabolises both relatively quickly and efficiently. But when it comes to fat it's a different story. Over thousands of years we humans have had to cope with times of hunger and shortage, and so our bodies evolved to become capable of hanging on to fat as a means of carrying us through the lean times between harvests, or when for other reasons food was scarce. It's only in relatively recent generations that we've been able to rely on getting enough food at any time. Our bodies may need a few more thousand years to 'learn' we don't need to store fat in the same way. Result? It's very easy to become overweight.

Not only do we store fat when we really don't need to, we also eat it when we don't need to. The Medical Research Council in Cambridge has done a lot of work with diet, weight and appetite, and has shown that fat simply doesn't fill us very well – so we end up eating more than we really need just to satisfy our hunger. We simply don't realise when we've had enough.

In one study, nutritionists tested the effects of secretly manipulating the diet of a group of men. Some men were given a diet which consisted of 20 per cent fat (that is, 20 per cent of the calories came from fat) and others were given a diet which consisted of 60 per cent fat. The amounts of food were not controlled and they were asked to eat according to appetite. The men on both diets ended up eating the same amount of food, with similar portions and frequency, but those on the 20 per cent diet lost 200g of body fat per week, while the 60 per centers gained 700g of fat per week. The reason was that the 60 per centers did not know when they'd had enough. Their diets did not issue 'stop eating' signals. This phenomenon is known as 'passive over-consumption'.

When the experiment was repeated with men who were more physically active, the differences between the 20 and 60 per centers were nothing like so great. This shows that physical exercise can work to counteract the ill-effects of a high-fat diet, and that the ideal healthy regime is a diet that is low in fat *and* high in activity.

Note: None of this means that fat in your diet is bad for you. We all need a certain amount of fat – but far less of the saturated fat that we tend to favour. Better for health are the polyunsaturated and monounsaturated oils from plants, nuts and seeds.

Cholesterol Explained

The link between cholesterol and heart disease has been well-established for a generation, but newer research has shown that we shouldn't be quick to condemn all cholesterol.

Cholesterol is a fat, needed throughout the body (though not built up on artery walls) as a vital constituent of cell membranes, the nervous system and important biochemicals. It is transported round the body by lipoproteins in the blood. HDLs, or high-density lipoproteins, act as scavengers of cholesterol and carry it away from tissues where it's no longer wanted (like on the arterial walls), to the liver. LDLs, or low-density lipoproteins, transport cholesterol from the liver to the rest of the body, including the arterial walls. Having HDL and LDL in balance is vital to cardiovascular health (the health of your heart and blood circulation system). Too high a level of LDL and you increase the risk of disease. High HDL levels are, however, generally good, and have been shown to be preventative of stroke and coronary heart disease.

A healthy diet, as outlined in this chapter and elsewhere in the book, maintains and can even restore the balance of HDLs and LDLs.

Garlic is Good News

Garlic has a reputation that stretches back centuries and is shared by many cultures. More recently, its power has been demonstrated by scientists and nutritionists, who are now convinced that it can do a lot more for you than flavour garlic bread and salad dressing!

Fruit and Vegetables

The current advice from the UK Department of Health is to eat five portions of fruit and vegetables a day. But what's a 'portion'? Here's what the advice is based on:

Vegetables (raw, cooked, frozen or canned) – 2 table-spoons
Salad – 1 dessert bowlful
Grapefruit/avocado pear – half a fruit
Apples, bananas, oranges – 1 fruit
Plums – 2 fruits
Grapes, cherries, berries – 1 cupful
Dried fruit – half to one tablespoonful
Fruit juice – 150 ml glass
Fresh fruit salad, stewed or canned fruit – 2–3 table-spoons (including a little juice or syrup)

Source: Health Education Authority

Do You Need Supplements?

Everything we need to stay healthy could come from our daily diet, but many of us have problems in getting every-thing regularly. Time may be short so we skip meals, fresh, good quality foods may not be available at all times, and we can't always keep a close eye on the nutrient content of what we eat.

Should You 'Go Organic'?

Organic foods – the term usually applies to cereals, fruit and vegetables – have been grown in healthy soil that hasn't been artificially changed by the addition of chemicals and hasn't been treated with synthetic pesticides or hormones or other substances. If you see meat labelled 'organic', it should mean that the animal from which it comes from has been reared non-intensively, allowed to roam, and fed on a diet free from chemicals and antibiotics.

There is no doubt that the nutritional value of foods can be affected by modern, non-organic ways of farming and organic foods may taste better, too. But whether choosing organic foods means you can make a crucial difference to your health is a controversial matter. The jury, as it were, is still out and proof one way or the other is very hard to come by.

Organic food is more widely available than it used to be, so it's easier than it was to make a choice. It still tends to be more expensive, however, because the smaller quantities grown mean higher overheads.

By plugging gaps in your diet, which may well be beneficial for your long-term health, supplements can be thought of as an insurance policy. They help you remain confident that your body is getting the nutrients it needs even on days when you aren't eating as well as you'd like. Doctors Reg Saynor and Frank Ryan, authors of *The Eskimo Diet*, for example, say that a daily portion of oily fish rules out the need for supplements, but people who eat fewer than two oily fish meals a week benefit from a daily 5 ml teaspoon or equivalent of fish oil supplement.

In addition the Government's National Food Survey recently revealed the importance of vitamins and minerals in the diet.

Angela and Supplements

'I take Seven Seas cod liver oil*, evening primrose oil* and ginseng* daily,' says Angela Rippon. 'They were originally recommended by a friend who always seemed extremely fit and well. I try to keep to a good healthy diet and manage to most of the time. But I feel the supplements I take are important as a back-up.'

* Cod liver oil contains a concentration of the important Omega 3 fatty acids that help maintain heart health and keep joints supple and flexible. Also a good natural source of vitamins A and D.
* Evening primrose oil is used by many people to maintain a healthy-looking skin, and it's also a good source of essential fatty acids. Some women take it to maintain hormonal balance.
* Many people believe ginseng helps maintain good health and vitality and is popular with many people who lead active and demanding lives.

The Menopause – A Real 'Change of Life'?

During and after the menopause, the ovaries stop producing the hormones oestrogen and progesterone. Not everyone finds this a problem, but those women who do have symptoms that are in part caused by the fall-off in these hormones.

HRT (hormone replacement therapy), which is prescribed to replace the 'missing' hormones, can help. However, it's not suitable for everyone because of side-effects which include anxiety and depression. Some women simply prefer not to take it, as they are concerned about research which shows an increase in the risk of some cancers in women who have been taking HRT (though research also shows a possible reduction in the risk of developing heart disease). Your doctor will discuss the pros and cons with you.

You can help stay healthy in later years by re-evaluating your diet.

Alcohol: Keep It Low

Current recommendations for a safe alcohol limit are two to three units a day for women and three to four units a day for men.

One unit of alcohol equals:

100 ml glass of wine
50 ml glass of sherry
25 ml measure of spirit – that's the usual pub measure
300 ml glass (half a pint) of normal strength beer

Chapter Ten

Your 14-Day Eating Plan

Definitely Not a 'Diet' – More a Change of Eating!

You *can* make changes to your diet, and the diet of anyone you buy and cook for. The rest of this book gives you plenty of ideas on what changes to make, and advises on foods you need to cut down on and the ones you can eat more of. This chapter is concerned with some suggestions on how to put it all into practice.

Healthy eating is best seen as a way of life, not as a quick fix to be abandoned after just a few weeks. But unless you have specific allergies or food intolerances, you don't have to rule out any foods for ever – occasional treats or indulgences on special occasions are not going to harm you.

If you have a real craving for some foods, however, such as those foods high in sugar or fats, like sweets, cakes or biscuits, it can be worth considering cutting them out completely if you really can't cut down. You may be one of those people who can't rest knowing there's a packet of biscuits or a chocolate bar in the cupboard – and trying to eat one biscuit at a time or just one square of chocolate is simply too difficult! But once you've gone through a couple of weeks of not having the food you crave, you will find the edge goes off your longing. You may even be able to have the food from time to time without bingeing on it.

Our suggested eating plan takes 14 days to complete. We don't expect you to stick to it rigidly – no one's life is that organised for that long! However, the closer you get to matching it, the healthier your diet. Of course, our ideas are only one of many different routes you can take to full nutritional fitness. You'll want to adapt your own ideas, along with ours, to suit your life, your family's preferences and the time you have available to shop and prepare.

Our programme works like this: we have suggested 14 different breakfasts, 14 different lunches and 14 different main meals. All the ideas are simple, use only a few ingredients and are manageable by even novice or average cooks – we haven't chosen anything that needs complicated preparation. You can of course combine any of the breakfasts with any of the other meals and swap a lunch for a main meal whenever you prefer.

The diet will help you lose weight if you have been eating more than you need up until now, but it is not specifically a 'slimming' diet. We don't give you precise ideas of quantity with this eating programme – the portions you eat will depend on your appetite. However, if you are keen to lose weight, you may want to control the size of your meals, and if you eat between meals, you should stick to low-calorie, low-fat snacks.

We haven't included details of drinks with this programme, but you should aim to drink several glasses of water a day, as that's good for keeping your system 'flushed through'. If you drink tea or coffee, try to have no more than four cups (of tea *and* coffee) a day. Instead, drink herbal or fruit teas. If you drink alcohol, stick to the limits on page 110. Don't drink highly sweetened soft drinks and remember diet drinks may be low in sugar, but they are often high in additives (colourings and flavourings). Fruit juice, diluted with water if you want a long drink, is healthier.

On page 118, you'll find recipes for many of the dishes mentioned.

Breakfasts

Always eat breakfast. Apart from the fact your body needs it, having gone all night with no food at all, skipping breakfast, or eating an inadequate breakfast, means you will feel ravenously hungry mid-morning and head for something instantly comforting but not necessarily nutritious. Have a small glass of fruit juice with your breakfast.

Here are some breakfast ideas:

1. Porridge, made with water or a mix of skimmed milk and water, and sweetened as lightly as you can, just enough to make it palatable. A wholemeal bread bun or one slice of wholemeal bread or toast with a minimum amount of butter, margarine or low-fat spread. Small amount of jam or marmalade if liked.
2. Wholegrain commercial breakfast cereal with skimmed milk. Fresh grapefruit or grapefruit segments from a can (choose the sort in its own juice). Bread/toast as before.
3. Poached or grilled kippers. Bread/toast as before.
4. Small can of baked beans served on wholemeal toast.
5. Soft boiled egg with bread/toast as before.
6. Home-made muesli (see recipes). Note we suggest you soak it the night before in skimmed milk and then add a topping of fruit like fresh orange segments or

sliced banana.

7. Wholemeal cereal served with warmed skimmed milk and topped with some dried fruit. Bread/toast as before.

8. Bought waffles, grilled or warmed, served with a drizzle of honey.

9. Carton of low-fat yoghurt mixed with a tinned or fresh pear and a tablespoon of crushed nuts (almonds taste best). Bread/toast as before.

10. Scrambled egg mixed with a small amount of skimmed milk served on bread or toast.

11. Oat cereal with skimmed milk or yoghurt, mixed with dried fruit. Bread/toast as before.

12. Mix a ripe banana, a teaspoonful of desiccated coconut, a handful of ground walnuts and some sesame seeds plus a small amount of skimmed milk in the blender.

13. Poached egg served on a slice of wholemeal toast.

14. Dried fruit (raisins, apricots, sultanas) soaked overnight in enough water to cover, with a handful of sesame seeds. Serve with Greek yoghurt and honey.

Lunches

Many of our lunches are centred on sandwiches – great nutritional value, especially if you use good quality ingredients and good bread. The bread doesn't always have to be wholegrain if you're getting fibre from other parts of your diet. Choose fillings with a variety of textures and tastes to keep up your interest. If you use butter or another spread, spread it thinly.

1. Tuna sandwiches with iceberg lettuce. Two satsumas or a piece of citrus fruit.

2. Mashed tinned sardines in tomato sauce grilled on a slice of bread or a bun, topped with sliced tomato. Low-fat fruit yoghurt.

3. Cottage cheese with chopped cucumber in a quarter of a baguette. Banana.

4. Cold chopped cooked chicken in low-fat mayonnaise with salad in a sandwich. Fresh fruit salad with ground almonds or walnuts sprinkled on the top.

5. Baked beans with sliced tomato on top served on toast. Grapefruit segments and Greek yoghurt.

6. Mashed pilchards on toast, with a few grilled mushrooms and a side salad. Apple.

7. Carton of low-fat coleslaw salad with lettuce, cucumber and tomato, a few raisins and sesame seeds, stuffed into pitta bread pocket. Fruit.

8. Carrot soup *(see recipes)* with roll. Orange and grapefruit segments with honey to taste.

9. Baked potato (quickly done in a microwave oven) with tuna and low-fat mayonnaise plus a salad. Fruit.

10. Grill a small pizza base covered with ketchup or tomato paste, three or four anchovies or sardines, sliced mushroom and grated or thinly sliced mozzarella cheese. Fromage frais.

11. Ham sandwich (cut off any visible fat on the sliced ham) with mustard and salad. Fruit.

12. Vegetable soup *(see recipes)*. Bread. Low-fat fruit yoghurt.

13. Chopped cooked turkey and salad in sandwich. Fromage frais.

14. Smoked mackerel pâté *(see recipes)* in a sandwich served with a side salad. Fruit.

Main Meals

Most of the meal suggestions here are served with a salad as it's such a useful and easy-to-prepare source of fresh, uncooked vegetables. You can make a quick, substantial salad from grated raw vegetables such as carrot or cabbage.

If you use a dressing on your salad, don't drown it! If it's an oil-based dressing, use a good quality olive oil. You can also add interest and texture to your salads, as well as give them a nutritional boost, by sprinkling ground or flaked nuts and/or seeds on top – sesame seeds, sunflower seeds and pumpkin seeds, for example, are all easily available in health stores, delicatessens and larger supermarkets. Remember, nuts and seeds are useful for their essential fatty acids.

1. Steak (grilled), baked or boiled potatoes, salad, broccoli. Baked apple and low-fat ice cream.
2. Chicken and vegetable casserole with mashed potato, mangetout peas, salad. Fresh fruit salad.
3. Ratatouille *(see recipes)* with rice. Frozen strawberries and/or raspberries drizzled with honey.
4. Grilled mackerel with gooseberry sauce *(see recipes)*, steamed chopped vegetables (peppers, mushrooms, beansprouts), boiled potatoes. Fruit vol-au-vents *(see recipes)*.
5. Seafood risotto *(see recipes)*, salad. Purchased fruit sorbet (from the frozen food compartment).
6. Tofu stir-fry with strips or squares of tofu, bean sprouts, mushrooms, chopped peppers, sweetcorn, carrot, etc. (a frozen bag of ready-prepared chopped vegetables is handy). Fromage frais.

7. Baked trout sprinkled with flaked almonds, boiled potatoes, salad, French beans. Ice cream mashed with banana.
8. Lasagne, salad. Fruit granita *(see recipes)*.
9. Roast chicken or turkey, green vegetables, carrots, dry roast potatoes *(see recipes)*. Purchased low-fat dessert.
10. Tofu and cauliflower crumble *(see recipes)*, salad, boiled potatoes. Fruit.
11. Spaghetti bolognese (use best-quality minced beef, as cheaper mince is high in fat), salad. Fresh fruit jelly.
12. Pasta with a quick sauce made of a purchased mushroom pasta sauce with strips of smoked salmon added. Fruit.
13. Fish pie (use any white fish), grilled after cooking with tomatoes on the top, salad, tinned peas. Fruit crumble.
14. Spanish omelette, made with eggs, diced vegetables (cooked potatoes, pepper, courgette). Green vegetable, such as French beans. Salad. Frozen yoghurt.

Recipes

All these quantities serve four people.

Carrot Soup

450g carrots, finely sliced
50g ground almonds
half pint skimmed or semi-skimmed milk
seasoning
parsley

Place all the ingredients except the parsley in a liquidiser or food processor and blend. Heat gently in a pan – don't boil. Add parsley when serving.

Fruit Granita

250ml sparkling white wine
250g frozen or fresh soft fruit

Mix together in a bowl, crushing the fruit without pulping it. Freeze overnight. Take out of the freezer about 10 minutes before serving to allow for some softening.

Fruit Vol-au-Vents

12 vol-au-vent cases
1 jar apple sauce
100g raisins
brandy to taste
fresh cream or crème fraiche
cinnamon

Soak the raisins in brandy for an hour and then add to the apple sauce, warming the mixture in a pan. Spoon into vol-au-vent cases. Serve with cream or *crème fraiche.* Sprinkle with cinnamon.

Grilled Mackerel with Gooseberry Sauce

Four mackerel, fresh or frozen
250g gooseberries, fresh or frozen
honey to sweeten

If you buy the fish from a fishmonger, ask for them to be trimmed and cleaned. Place on a piece of foil and grill under a medium heat until cooked (about 5 to 10 minutes, depending on size). Add the fruit to an inch of water in a pan and cook for about five minutes on a medium heat until softened. Blend with the honey in a liquidiser. Serve with the mackerel, reheating first.

Home-Made Muesli

2 cups of porridge oats
1 tablespoon of wheatgerm (commercially available as Bemax)
1 tablespoon golden linseeds
2 cups of skimmed or semi-skimmed milk
2 tablespoons of dried mixed fruit
2 tablespoons of ground hazelnuts
1 tablespoon desiccated coconut

Soak overnight in the fridge. Add warmed milk if liked the next morning in order to moisten to taste. Add chopped fresh fruit on serving.

Ratatouille

250g chopped aubergines
250g chopped courgettes
1 each of red, green and yellow peppers, chopped
250g onions, sliced
400g can tomatoes
2 cloves of garlic, crushed
1 tablespoon of tomato purée
2 tablespoons olive oil
seasoning

Heat the oil and add the aubergines. After five minutes or so over a medium heat add the courgettes, then the onions and peppers. Heat the tomatoes, garlic and tomato purée in another pan and simmer for three to five minutes until reduced slightly. Sieve and add to the other pan. Simmer for 10 to 15 minutes until the vegetables are cooked.

Seafood Risotto

300g fresh fish, any type
2 onions, chopped
500g cooked rice
250g frozen prawns
small can peas
2 tablespoons olive oil
chopped chives
seasoning

Grill fish for 5 to 10 minutes, depending on size, until
cooked. Flake into pieces. Lightly fry the onion in a pan
and add the fish, prawns, rice and can of peas. Stir well
for several minutes – check prawns are softened and mix
is heated through. Season to taste. Garnish with
chopped chives on serving.

Smoked Mackerel Pâté

250g smoked mackerel fillet, skinned and flaked
100g plain cottage cheese
juice of half a lemon
1 teaspoon horseradish sauce
seasoning

Mix all the ingredients in a blender. Put the mixture into
a bowl and refrigerate overnight.

Tofu and Cauliflower Crumble

250g chopped leeks
1 small onion
half a white cabbage, chopped
three quarters of a pint of stock (or chicken or vegetable stock
cube made with water)
200g tofu, chopped
medium cauliflower, broken into florets
200g toasted breadcrumbs (grill breadcrumbs for a few seconds
under a hot grill, on foil)
seasoning
2 tablespoons olive oil

Heat the oil, add the chopped leeks and the chopped onion and cook over a medium heat for about five minutes. Add the cabbage and stock and bring to the boil. Simmer for 5 to 10 minutes. Meanwhile steam the cauliflower for five minutes in another pan. Add the tofu to the cabbage pan and cook for a further five minutes. Bring contents of both pans together in a baking dish and season to taste. Top with toasted breadcrumbs.

Vegetable Soup

1 medium onion, chopped
2 cloves garlic, crushed
2 sticks celery, chopped
2 carrots, chopped
250g tomatoes, skinned
can of beans (for example, cannellini, butter, kidney)
1½ pints of stock
2 tablespoons olive oil
seasoning

Heat the oil and soften the onion and the garlic in it. Add the remaining vegetables (except the can of beans) and stir well. Add stock and seasoning, and quickly bring to the boil. Cover and simmer for about 20 minutes. Stir in the can of beans and heat through for a further two to three minutes.

Section Four

STAY IN TOUCH

Chapter Eleven
Get Organised!

Here's our jam-packed guide to organisations, information and support you might find useful for yourself or your friends. We've included the addresses of some of the sports and activities organisations you might find valuable. They can tell you about training courses, facilities and events going on in your area.

We've also borne in mind that many older people have caring responsibilities for partners, friends or parents. Some of the sources here will be useful as sources of information on benefits and practical help with day-to-day care. Some of these organisations have special helplines offering on-the-spot advice. Turn to our helplines section for a selection of telephone contacts for instant guidance and information.

For your Address Book

Age Concern
Astral House
1268 London Road
London SW16 4ER
Telephone: 0181-679 8000

The UK's largest charity providing direct services to older people.

Alexander Technique International
142 Thorpdale Road
London N4 3BS
Telephone: 0171-281 7639

Send a stamped self-addressed A5 envelope for a list of teachers.

Alzheimer's Disease Society
Gordon House
10 Greencoat Place
London SW1P 1PH
Telephone: 0171-306 0606

Support and information for people suffering from Alzheimer's Disease and other dementias, and their carers. The society has local branches in all parts of the country.

The Amateur Swimming Association
Harold Fem House
Derby Square
Loughborough
Leicestershire
LE11 0AL
Telephone: 01509 230431

The Arthritic Association
First Floor Suite
2 Hyde Gardens
Eastbourne
BN21 4PN
Telephone: 0171-491 0233

Dietary guidance and information on complementary treatment for arthritis.

Arthritis and Rheumatism Council for Research
PO Box 177
Chesterfield
Derbyshire
S41 7TQ
Telephone: 01246 558033

ASH (Action on Smoking and Health)
Devon House
11–15 Dartmouth Street
London SW1H 9BL
Telephone: 0171-314 1360

Information on giving up smoking, including developing workplace policies. ASH can refer to local support groups.

Association of Crossroads Care Attendant Schemes
10 Regent Place
Rugby
Warwickshire
CV21 2PN
Telephone: 01788 573653

Crossroads Care schemes offer a befriending and respite care service to carers and their relatives.

BACUP (British Association of Cancer United Patients)
3 Bath Place
Rivington Street
London EC2A 3JR
Telephone: 0171-696 9003

Founded by cancer patients, BACUP offers up-to-date advice and information on treatment options and on self-help for all types of cancer.

The Badminton Association of England
National Badminton Centre
Bradwell Road
Loughton Lodge
Milton Keynes
Buckinghamshire
MK8 9LA
Telephone: 01908 568822

Bristol Cancer Help Centre
Grove House
Cornwallis Grove
Bristol BS8 4PG
Telephone: 0117 980 9500

Information on conventional and complementary therapies, dietary advice and residential stays at this famous centre.

The British Allergy Foundation
St Bartholomew's Hospital
London EC1A 7BE
Telephone: 0171-600 6127

Research and information about allergies of all types for
medical specialist and the public.

The British Diabetic Association
10 Queen Anne Street
London W1M OBD
Telephone: 0171-323 1531

Information on diabetes and support for research into
the condition.

The British Heart Foundation
14 Fitzhardinge Street
London W1H 4DH
Telephone: 0171-935 0185

Raises money for research and offers information to
patients; promotes good heart health.

The British Wheel of Yoga
1 Hamilton Placc
Boston Road
Sleaford
Lincolnshire
NG34 7ES
Telephone: 01529 306851

Send a stamped self-addressed envelope for a factsheet
and information about teachers.

Carers' National Association
Ruth Pitter House
20–25 Glasshouse Yard
London EC1A 4JS
Telephone: 0171-490 8818

For all people with caring responsibilities.

Counsel and Care
Twyman House
16 Bonny Street
London NW1 9PG
Telephone: 0171-485 1566

Free advice for older people and their families, with published factsheets on issues such as benefits, accommodation and help at home.

Cruse Bereavement Care
Cruse House
126 Sheen Road
Richmond
Surrey
TW9 1UR
Telephone: 0181-940 4818

Counselling and support for people who are bereaved.

Disabled Living
4 St Chad's Street
Manchester M8 8QA
Telephone: 0161-832 3678

Information and support on living with a disability; also

information on household and independent care aids.

Exercise Association of England
Unit 4
Angel Gate
326 City Road
London EC1V 2PT
Telephone: 0171-278 0811

Call for details of qualified exercise teachers in your area.

Exodus Biking Adventures
9 Weir Road
London SW12 0LT
Telephone: 0181-673 0859

See page 142.

The Health Education Authority
Hamilton House
Mabledon Place
London WC1H 9TX
Telephone: 0171-413 1987

National information centre on preventive health, diet, alcohol, smoking and other major health topics.

The Lawn Tennis Association
The Queens Club
Barons Court
London W14 9EG
Telephone: 0171-381 7000

The National Association for Colitis and Crohn's Disease
4 Beaumont House
Sutton Road
St Albans
Hertfordshire
AL1 5HH
Telephone: 01727 844296

Dietary and other advice and information for sufferers of these two conditions.

The National Back Pain Association
16 Elm Tree Road
Teddington
Middlesex
TW11 8ST
Telephone: 0181-977 5474

Information and research for sufferers of all types of back pain.

The National Heart Research Fund
Concord House
Park Lane
Leeds LS3 1EQ
Telephone: 0113 234 7474

Campaigns for better education about healthier lifestyles; raises money for research; offers support to patients and families.

The National Osteoporosis Society
PO Box 10
Radstock
Bath
BA3 3YB
Telephone: 01761 471771

Research into the treatment and prevention of this disease, and support for sufferers.

The Open University
P0 Box 200
Walton Hall
Milton Keynes
MK7 6YZ
Telephone: 01908 653231

Write or call for details of courses *(see page 141)*.

The Patients' Association
8 Guildford Street
London WC1N 1DT
Telephone: 0171-242 3460

Campaigns for views of patients to be heard.

QUIT
Victory House
170 Tottenham Court Road
London W1P OHA
Telephone: 0171-388 5775

Help for people who want to stop smoking.

The Ramblers' Association
1–5 Wandsworth Road
London SW8 2XX
Telephone: 0171-582 6878

Ramblers' Holidays
Box 43
Welwyn Garden
AL8 6PQ
Telephone: 01707 331133

See page 142.

The Shiatsu Society
Interchange Studios
Dalby Street
London NW5 3NQ
Telephone: 0171-813 7772

Send a stamped self-addressed envelope for a list of
teachers.

The Stroke Association
CHSA House
123 Whitecross Street
London EC1 8JJ
Telephone: 0171-490 7999

For people who have suffered a stroke and their relatives.

The University of the Third Age (U3A)
26 Harrison Street
London WC1H 8JG
Telephone: 0171-837 8838

See page 141.

The Veteran Squash Racket Club of Great Britain
Summertrees
27 Leatherhead Road
Leatherhead
Surrey
KT22 8TL
Telephone: 01442 232222

Women's Health Concern
93/103 Upper Richmond Road
London SW15 2TG
Telephone: 0181-780 3007

Information and awareness-raising on all aspects of women's health, including the menopause and hormone replacement therapy.

Telephone Helplines

These numbers are all special helplines for the public. Not all are open 24 hours a day, but most should have an answering message telling you of access hours.

BACUP – 0800 18 11 99
(See entry above.)

Benefit Enquiry Line – 0800 88 22 00
For disabled people and their carers.

Benefits Agency Freeline – 0800 666 555
For advice on all benefits and national insurance contributions.

Breast Cancer Care – 0500 245 345
For people who have breast cancer or fear they may have breast cancer, plus their families.

Cancerlink – 0171-833 2451
For people with any form of cancer or their families.

Carers' National Association – 0171-490 888
(See entry above.)

Counsel and Care Advice Line – 0171-485 1586
(See entry above.)

Cruse Bereavement Line – 0181-332 7227
(See entry above.)

DIAL UK – 01302 310123
The national HQ of the DIAL network of disability advice services.

Disability Alliance Rights Line – 0171-247 8763
For disabled people and their carers.

Drinkline – 0345 320202
Advice and information for anyone concerned about their own or someone else's drinking.

First Steps to Freedom – 01926 851608
For people who suffer general anxiety, including people who are coming off tranquillisers, and their families.

Heartline – 0800 85 85 85
Information about heart disease, prevention and treatment.

MIND – 0345 660163
Information about mental health and treatment and services for people who are mentally ill and their families.

The Mobility Information Service – 01743 761889
For the physically disabled who wish to drive or to return to driving after illness or disablement.

The National Osteoporosis Society – 01761 472721
(See entry above.)

Pain Concern – 01227 264677
For chronic pain sufferers and their family and friends.

The Samaritans – 0345 90 90 90
For anyone in distress.

SANELINE – 0345 67 8000
For anyone coping with mental illness.

Senior Line – 0800 65 00 65
Information on issues of concern to older people and their families, including accommodation, welfare and benefits.

Women's Health Concern – 0181-556 1966
(See entry above.)

Women's Nationwide Cancer Control Campaign – 0171-729 2229
For women and their families concerned about issues relating to cancer screening, especially breast and cervical cancer.

Chapter Twelve
New Interests, New Ideas

Here are some activities and interests you may not have tried before, some geared especially to the needs of older people. They may give you some new ideas!

If you are already retired, you can join the University of the Third Age – or U3A, as it's known. U3A has groups all over the country, dedicated to the notion of staying fit mentally as well as physically. It offers plenty of social opportunities as well, with events organised for groups throughout the year, usually involving walking, keep fit and swimming, but there are non-physical activities, too, as members themselves choose the programme. There are over 300 groups at present, with 50,000 members. *See page 137 for a contact address.*

The Open University offers educational and training opportunities to thousands of people of all ages – some students are in their 80s and 90s. You don't just work for a degree, as there are many more qualifications on offer. Most courses offer a combination of home-based study with outside lectures and seminars, often held over a residential weekend or longer. *Address on page 135.*

Active holidays with a difference make a change from lounging around soaking up the sun! The National Trust has a range of working and skills-based holidays on which you can learn about crafts and tasks such as dry-stone walling, forestry, falconry and other country pursuits. Or what about signing up for a working holiday with the British Trust for Conservation Volunteers? You can contribute with your muscle and energy to conservation and environmental projects in all areas of the country, and enjoy working as a member of a like-minded team.

If you're interested in walking holidays, gentle, not so gentle, at home or in the most exotic locations abroad, contact Ramblers' Holidays *(address page 136)* who've been organising walks anywhere and everywhere for 50 years.

Cycling holidays are becoming more and more adventurous – and there are a number of specialist operators. For one offering a wide choice try Exodus Biking Adventures, who arrange trips lasting between one and three weeks both at home and abroad *(address page 133)*.

Don't forget the evening and afternoon classes on offer in every town and city as part of local adult education programmes. Universities and colleges also run part-time and short courses often open to all-comers. Maybe this is the year when you finally learn that foreign language, develop your wine-tasting skills, perfect your DIY skills, or whatever – if you want to learn it, there's a place you can do it!

Index